Hungry Woman

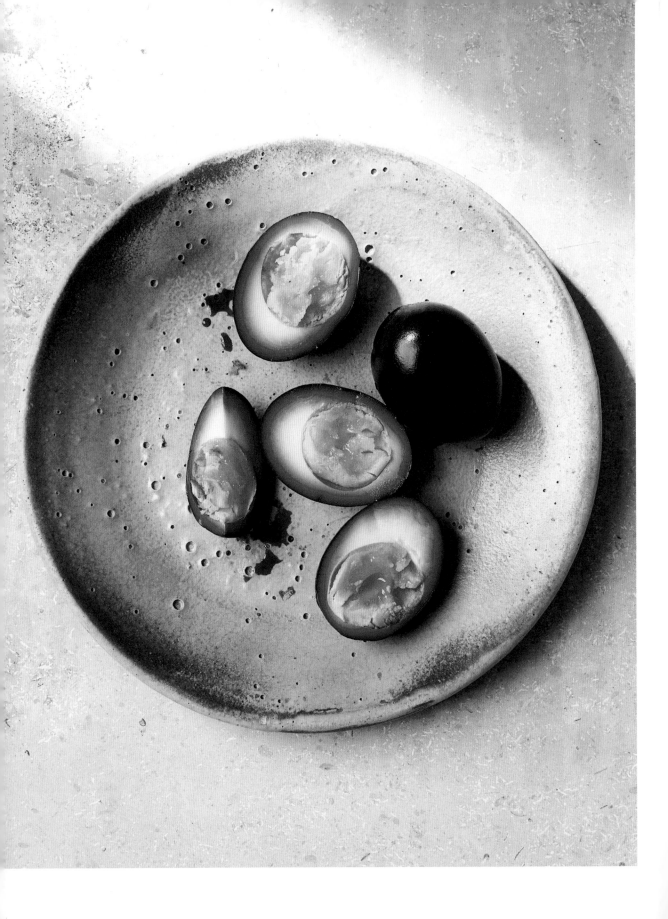

Eating for good health,
happiness + hormones

Pauline Cox, MSc
Foreword by
Julia Bradbury

Hungry Woman

EBURY
PRESS

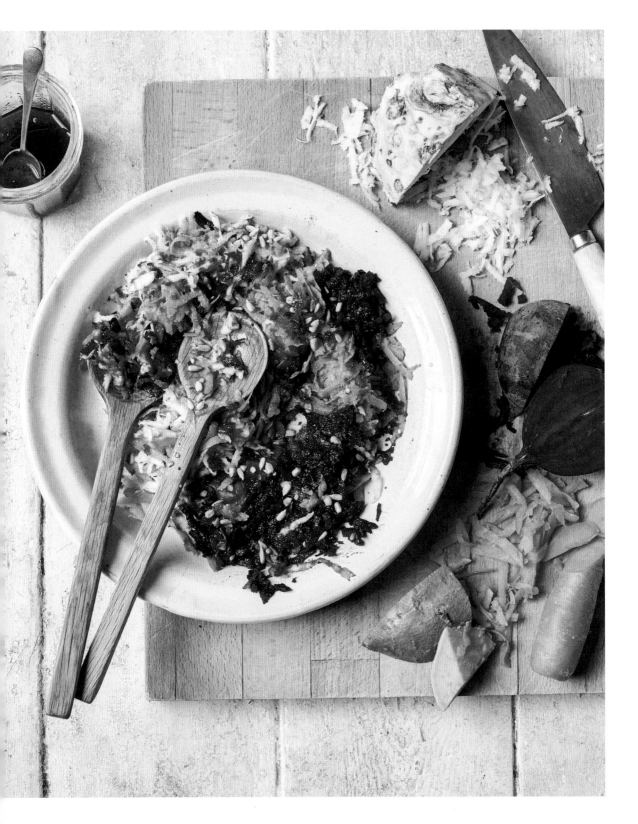

Raw slaw, recipe on page 154

CONTENTS

Foreword by Julia Bradbury

I always welcome a new book that discusses health and nutrition in a meaningful, informed way. Our health is taking a battering in the modern world; sedentary lifestyles, daily exposure to pollution and toxins, the relatively new 'never switch off' approach – all have a detrimental impact on our physical and mental health. Women's health, in particular, has been overlooked and under-researched for centuries, and the conversation has only just begun to gather traction, which in my opinion is utterly mad considering we make up half the population. In her brilliant book *Invisible Women*, Caroline Criado Perez exposes a world where, although women make up 50 per cent of the human race, men are used as the standard default to test almost everything, from product design to urban planning – in spite of our different societal roles and physiology. When it comes to medical matters, textbooks overwhelmingly use male bodies. Women are under-represented in clinical trials and comparatively little research has been done on ailments particular to women. Frustratingly, we continue to hear stories of doctors dismissing patients when they exhibit 'female symptoms' and 'women's issues'. It is not so long ago that physicians were keen to banish women to asylums for behaviour inconsistent with femininity.

When it comes to hormones and women's health, we have a long way to go, and I'm afraid to say our hormones are still getting in the way of medical progress! The fluctuating levels of hormones throughout a woman's menstrual cycle and lifespan have resulted in women historically being excluded from clinical trials. Female bodies have been perceived as too complicated and too costly to research.

This means that evidence gathered about the safety and effectiveness of medications doesn't apply to women: we metabolise them differently and our bodies are biologically different, right down to the cellular level. Lower body weight, slower digestion, less activity from intestinal enzymes and slower filtration by the kidneys are all factors that cause this difference. Medications can also have varying effects depending on the time they are taken in the menstrual cycle, as well as affecting the menstrual cycle itself. This lack of information leaves a dangerous knowledge gap that has a real impact on the safety of women within healthcare. Not surprisingly, a recent research study found that women experience up to twice as many adverse drug reactions as men.

So, we're different to men, require a different approach and more empathy and understanding when it comes to our needs. I believe we also need to learn and research as much information as we can about our own bodies, and to turn to each other for help and advice. Fortunately, there is a burgeoning number of female experts, nutritionists and physicians who are collecting more and more data and sharing their knowledge within the medical community at large and with us. Social media has also made sharing stories on forums easier and that can add valuable comfort – knowing that someone else is going through a similar experience. I'm not saying all male doctors don't understand us; but the statistics show that we need more representation, more studies and more women in key specialist roles. And we need to keep exploring new paths – like the impact of nutrition on our hormones.

While some of us may have been taught what to expect from our bodies during menstruation, we probably weren't informed about the hormonal fluctuations that affect the body throughout the entire month and throughout our lives. The decline in hormone production, progesterone and oestrogen for women and testosterone for men, is perhaps the most profound body chemistry change we go through in midlife. This process can begin as early as our late thirties and it doesn't only affect our body fat distribution, it can also lead to disrupted sleep, lower energy levels and mood swings. Diet can't replace these lost hormones but eating healthily will help support the endocrine system (the glands and organs that make hormones) generally, and there are certain foods that are known to be particularly beneficial for this.

Since my breast cancer diagnosis in 2021, I have taken a forensic interest in health and how nutrition and exercise can impact my hormones. I have focused my TV brain on stories about wellbeing, movement, longevity and stress management. Cortisol, which is known as the primary stress hormone alongside adrenaline (also known as epinephrine), plays a bigger role in our overall health than I ever gave it credit for. Balancing our two key sex hormones, oestrogen and progesterone, is crucially important for health. An imbalance of these sex hormones drives a number of symptoms that become accepted as part of 'being a woman'. Oestrogen dominance is a contributing factor to our risk of developing female cancers. Understanding the influence diet and lifestyle has on our hormones is an important means to living well and reducing our risk of chronic health issues.

As a woman, in the perimenopausal stage of life, I admit my awareness was limited and although I had a healthy-ish approach to life, it took something to go horribly wrong before I took a more proactive attitude. Now I am in awe of the beautiful and complicated web of body systems that work so brilliantly together, but I also understand a little more about how we need to help them along – and food alongside exercise are two of the most important levers we have. Our brains and our guts, our immune and respiratory systems, digestive tracts, blood vessels, skeletal structures, nervous and endocrine systems – all sing along with efficient intricacy. Unless a member of the orchestra starts to play out of tune. In this book you will learn the power of food to help fine tune the body.

I hope you find this book as fascinating and useful as I do, and that it helps you to better understand the power you have to influence your mood, sleep, weight, energy levels and overall wellbeing through simple dietary and lifestyle habits, in a more profound way that encourages you to maximise your health and hormones.

It's Time for Change ...

Forget the old concept that we have to live with the symptoms of hormonal disruption … we have normalised heavy and irregular periods, PMS, hormonal weight gain, fatigue and anxiety, brain fog, hot flushes and night sweats for too long!

Navigating the hormonal landscape from puberty, through to our later years in life may feel like a feat of ingenuity … however it is far simpler than you may think. As women, we are subject to hormonal challenges at all stages of our female lives, from the first flurry of hormones at puberty, to the more fertile years of our twenties and thirties. The perilous perimenopause can catch many women unaware before moving through to menopause and beyond.

Science is offering a far greater understanding of how the food we eat and the lifestyle choices we make can have a huge influence over our hormonal health. In this book, you will be guided to understand how the food choices you make on a daily basis impact your **hormonal balance**, **energy levels**, **sleep**, **weight status**, **mental wellbeing**, **focus**, **clarity of thought** and **overall wellbeing**.

This Book Will Guide You Through

UNDERSTANDING YOUR HORMONES

Identifying hormonal imbalances and WHY they are imbalanced. While hormones fluctuate and change throughout our females lives, they are exquisitely influenced by factors that are very much in our control. Learn how you can make simple changes to your diet and lifestyle to create BALANCED and HARMONIOUS hormones.

EATING FOR HORMONAL BALANCE

I have met thousands of women over my career as a Functional Nutritionist who feel incredibly frustrated when it comes to losing weight and eating well. When our metabolic and sex hormones are imbalanced, losing weight becomes a battle, often ending in frustration and self-loathing. When we work with our physiology, establishing an environment that allows the body to freely burn body fat, losing stubborn weight becomes a side-effect of eating and living well. In this book, you will learn that balancing your metabolic and sex hormones is a tasty and satisfying process!

NUTRIENT KNOW-HOW

A little nutrient know-how goes a long way! Which nutrients can improve my anxiety, hot flushes or painful periods … ? With so many supplements, powders and superfoods on the market, knowing which ones work and where to start can feel daunting! With two Bachelor's of Science, a Masters in Nutrition and Public Health and post-graduate training in Integrative Medicine, in this book I will provide the lowdown on supplements that can help support and alleviate symptoms and which foods offer you your best daily dose of nutrients.

MOUTH-WATERING MEALS … TO LEAVE YOU SATISFIED AND ENERGISED!

I know how addictive sugar is … I was gripped by its clutches for years. It was only when I learnt how to effectively burn my own body fat that I stopped being a slave to my metabolism and constant hunger, and at the mercy of hormonal havoc. I understand, I know the challenges … but liberating yourself from the vicious cycle of a poor relationship with food starts with giving your body what it needs, ditching the dieting and focusing on food that is packed with nutrients, flavour and satisfaction. In this book you will find 100 easy-to-follow recipes, that will leave you feeling fuelled and energised!

There is no need to live any longer with the frustration of hormonal imbalance … banish brain fog, ease anxiety and start living your best life with this straightforward, step-by-step guide on how to optimise and balance your metabolic and sex hormones.

Introduction

DISCOVERING YOU

This could arguably be one of the most important stories that you will ever read; it's the story of you – of how you work, what makes you function, what makes you tick … and what makes you sick.

The mysteries of your body will be revealed, and will challenge your current beliefs – those that have been drilled into you since childhood, which are unknowingly driving your daily decisions and the habits that see you buying a skinny caramel-mocha-chocca-frappé-latte over having boiled eggs for breakfast.

Even as you read this page, a synchronised series of biological messages is influencing every cell, tissue and system within your body. These biological messages form an internal coordinated communication system – your hormones.

At the most fundamental level, these potent hormonal cocktails are perfectly blended to drive you to carry out key actions that will ensure your survival – eat, have sex, have children, move. They motivate you, make you feel hungry, excited or aroused. Our hormones direct every aspect of our health, our energy levels, sex drive, fertility, mood, our body weight, muscle mass, hunger, satiety, our motivation, drive, sleep and relaxation. Even our experience of life, the relationship we have with our environment and with ourselves, is rooted in our hormones.

Disruption of our exquisite hormonal system is at the mercy of our modern lifestyle and diet, highly influenced by what we eat and drink, how we think, how we move, the stresses we experience, the levels of sunlight we are exposed to and the quality of our sleep. Hormone-disrupting dietary habits, lifestyle patterns and environmental influences have led to common hormonal imbalances that are now normalised and accepted as part of 'being a woman'.

In our uncertain, non-stop lives we have not only lost our connection with nature, but also with our own bodies. We no longer hear the whispers of our own biofeedback – such as heavy periods, low mood, insomnia and anxiety – instead, we normalise these symptoms as inconveniences we must manage, accept and live with.

Our hormones are affected by every aspect of our day-to-day lives, and our quality of life is hugely influenced and affected by our hormones! This bi-directional relationship can be confusing to even the most experienced of endocrinologists, and science is still untangling the intricacies of the inner crosstalk of our hormones and the powerful impact they have on all aspects of our health and wellbeing.

Recognising and correcting hormonal imbalances is a lot easier than living with them, and that starts with a little biology 101. Getting to know your body, understanding that the actions you take on a minute-by-minute basis are influencing your hormonal harmony – from what you choose to eat to when you choose to eat it. These decisions have a cumulative impact on your hormones as you travel through the hormonal timeline of your female lifespan. It is never too early or too late to think about balancing your hormones.

Our hormones are under attack! OK, that sounds a little dramatic, however our hormones are constantly being shunted and shifted as a result of our daily choices – how we live, the stress we experience, the food choices we make, the toxins we are exposed to, the amount of sleep we have. Our hormones are at the mercy of modern living and these shifts have a major impact on the quality of our lives from the moment we enter our teenage years right through to our post-menopausal period. Our hormones play crucial roles at every checkpoint in our lives, from their erratic explosion onto the party scene at puberty to the neuroprotective effects of oestrogen as we age.

Addressing hormonal imbalances first starts with an understanding of how the day-to-day choices we make can unwittingly upset the perfect dance between our key sex hormones, oestrogen and progesterone. Understanding how our diet and lifestyle choices impact our menstrual cycle can offer valuable clues to our hormonal status. Learning how to 'read' our periods from the colour of our menstrual blood to the heaviness, and the flow, can give an insight into our hormone health. How we live and the food we eat can powerfully influence fertility, PMS, weight status, mental wellbeing and the symptoms of perimenopause and menopause, governed by our fluctuating hormones.

With a greater understanding of our own bodies, we can reduce the suffering many women experience and accept as we transition through our hormonal lifespan, from puberty to our fertile years and from perimenopause to menopause and beyond.

Having a hold of our hormonal health, feeling in control and in flow with the cyclical changes we experience on a month-by-month basis provides peace of mind and serves as an invaluable source of feedback from the body. It is extremely challenging to be optimally heathy when our hormones are out of balance, and our bodies tell us one way or another when that's the case. Just like the language of chemical signals directed from the brain to the glands and tissues of the body, the symptoms of imbalance can be read, interpreted and corrected. Understanding our hormones, and their influence on our immediate and long-term health, liberates us from the confusion and frustration of changing body shapes, resistant weight gain, hair loss, low mood, low sex drive, anger, rage, depression and all the many emotional and physical changes that accompany the changing hormonal landscape, not just on a monthly basis, but over our lifespans.

This book is for all women of all ages, to help untangle and simplify the confusion of hormonal health. Getting to grips with how our monthly cycles influence our mood, mental state, our cravings and nutritional needs. How our hormones change over our female lifespan, from puberty, to perimenopause and beyond. It offers insights into the key hormone disruptors synonymous with modern life and how we can optimise hormonal balance with some key nutritional principles and lifestyle choices. It will cover common hormonal imbalances, why they happen and how we can re-establish hormonal harmony as well as an overview of hormonal changes over the female lifespan, from puberty to menopause. It will also cover the essential nutrients and supplements for building healthy hormones and the principles of a healthy diet for hormonal balance.

Some basic knowledge around your brain chemistry will give you a deeper understanding and insight into mood, anxiety, cravings and addictive behaviours that can see our best efforts to eat better thrown off track. Changing eating behaviours starts with balancing our brain chemistry as well as building a strong and resilient nervous system. In this book, you will be introduced to your neurotransmitters, a group of brain hormones that are highly influential on your eating habits and strong desires for certain foods. These powerful chemicals influence your mood, motivation, get-up-and-go, as well as feelings of calm. They govern many of the actions you take and the decisions you make on a daily basis. What you eat and how you live influences their levels within the brain. Learning how to optimise and balance our brain chemistry is hugely empowering, helping to liberate you from the clutches of cravings and bolster your motivation and feel-good hormones.

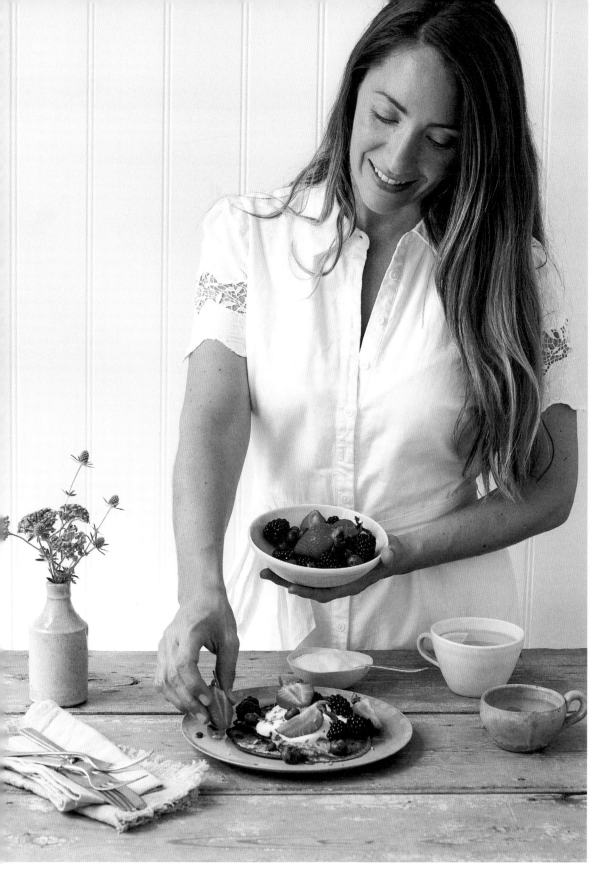

FROM SELF-MEDICATED TO SELF-DEDICATED

Finding freedom from exhaustion, poor sleep, low mood and lack of energy liberates you. It allows you to make choices and decisions from a place of feeling happy and in control. Choosing what to eat becomes a decision made based upon what you enjoy, what makes you feel good, what you love and what will love you back! You stop being a slave to your metabolism – instead, you start owning it.

When you're tired, anxious and too busy to think about what to eat, food becomes a frustration, a point of pain, but also a deep source of comfort. Self-medicating with sugar, caffeine and alcohol sees us driving ourselves to feel energised in the morning, only to wind down our over-stimulated minds in the evening with a glass or two of wine.

A deficiency in key nutrients can lead to biological systems within the body functioning at suboptimal levels. Our demanding brain for one, needs essential nutrients in order to function at the most fundamental level, firing up the communication between brain cells, lighting up our brain with ideas and possibilities, sparking creativity and forging memories. Building key brain hormones – neurotransmitters – in order to help us feel happy, alert, motivated, connected, relaxed or sleepy at appropriate times of the day. The energy-expensive task of running the brain alone demands we provide the boisterous brain with the nutrients needed … or risk the wrath of our hungry brain leaving us feeling tired, lethargic, low in mood and unmotivated.

Our energy levels and mood often drive our daily choices, whether we 'feel' like going for a morning stroll, power walk or gentle jog or heading off to the gym first thing, or simply rolling over and hitting snooze. This battle of wills can feel confusing, as one day you feel as committed, empowered and motivated as Mel Robbins, whipping yourself up with promises of new beginnings and fresh starts, while the next day your resolve disappears as quickly as your third coffee and custard cream.

Fear not … this journey does not come down to willpower and positive affirmations. Understanding old running narratives in our head is important, absolutely. However, no amount of motivational self-talk is going to spark up and energise your brain without the essential nutrients needed to fuel our hungry brains.

Setting the foundations for great health in place, building from a strong base where, yes, we may have the odd bad day and demolish the biscuits before dinner is even on the table … however those will be zigs on a long journey of zags. Building strong foundations of health will see your energy levels, mood AND motivation firmly set in place. There is no depriving yourself. This isn't about hiding the biscuit barrel and sitting on your hands. No! Far from feeling deprived, you will feel more fulfilled and satisfied that you ever thought possible.

**'Nothing in life is to be feared, it is only to be understood.
Now is the time to understand more, so that we may fear less.'**

— MARIE CURIE

In this book I encourage you to first spend a little time understanding your body, getting to know you and how you work. Why we get hormonal imbalances, excessive hunger, low energy or stubborn body fat. How we can help safeguard our health and longevity. It's only after we understand more that we can take action and empower ourselves with the solution.

So, are you ready?! Let's do this …

One

Accidently Unwell

'I used to recognise myself … how and when did my appearance change so much? Who is that person?' Catching your reflection unexpectedly in a shop window, finding yourself tagged in an unsuspected photo on a work night out, or simply seeing yourself as if for the first time in the bathroom mirror in the cold light of day; these bodies that we have become so comfortably accustomed to roaming around in suddenly become a surprisingly unfamiliar stranger. A running narrative starts questioning this case of stolen identity. Our bodies change shape – once-flexible limbs stiffen, our shapely trunks thicken like the trunk of a tree laying down concentric rings year upon year.

The real slap in the face is that it's not just our physicality that can become a stranger to us, but also the *person* inhabiting this unrecognisable body. Who is this tired, fatigued, anxious woman? When did my tolerance to the challenges of life become so short and snappy? Health struggles, aches and pains, migraines or sleep issues become the norm … but when did this happen? You can hardly remember the vibrant, youthful individual who once bounded through the day full of optimism, ideals and skinny jeans, brimming with hope and unbridled certainty that the world is there for the taking. You are left wondering … when exactly did I become accidentally unwell?

This is where I found myself a few months after giving birth to my second child. Having worked as a health professional for years, I prided myself on being a passionate advocate of a healthy diet and lifestyle and felt confident that I knew the choices I had been making were benefitting my health. However, I was becoming increasingly frustrated with what I felt was a blatant betrayal of my body. I was following my strong beliefs about what I *thought* was a healthy diet and the results of which were speaking for themselves. I was tired – all of the time. I leaned on the comfort of sugar to get me through the day, devouring biscuits only to be left feeling shameful and full of remorse when one quickly became ten. Hunger was a deep-set feeling that never really left, no matter how much I filled myself with stodgy carbs and sweets. No sooner had I felt the blissful sensation of sugar rushing through my body, I wanted more, I needed more, just to get through the day.

Hormonal issues had become something of a normality, with heavy periods, anaemia, bloating, carb cravings and stubborn weight gain. I felt as if I'd lost the person that I once was; the happy, vibrant, full-of-life individual that I had known for most of my adult life had not surfaced in some time. I knew she was in there, begging me to rescue her, to revive her, to breathe life back into the person I believed I was. My frustrations were amplified by the fact that I 'wanted' so much to be healthy, I just couldn't seem to find a way forward without being constantly drawn back to the habits I had become so familiar with.

Why did I feel so bad? Why did my body not feel like my own? Why could I not control the feelings of anger that could spring up at any given moment? The feelings of guilt for not being able to control my anger were a predictable follow on, all washed down with a healthy dose of exhaustion surmounted by a sense of failure that became my constant companion. The pain of living this way had become so insufferable that in the end it was the leverage I needed to seek out an alternative.

What if it wasn't me? What if this was down to more than willpower? What if my body needed something that it wasn't getting? Surely if I was giving my body everything it needed, I wouldn't feel this way? I knew my body had the innate intelligence to find balance, to find wellbeing, when it was provided with what was necessary for health. At that point, I didn't know what changes I needed to make, but I knew I had to make them.

I reassured myself that I would find the answer, that I would pull myself out of this rut. My struggle would become my strength. I knew I would find a better way of serving myself so that I could once again thrive and restore the energy that I so desperately wanted to feel, waking me up to life again.

I did what I knew best – I researched, I read and I scanned for answers. I looked at what I was doing at the time – eating a vegetarian diet, packed with carbohydrates, oats, grains, brown rice, dates, anything sweet that I could dress up as 'healthy'. Then it dawned on me that I was a complete sugar addict. I started looking to my cellular physiology for guidance, to understand what my body fundamentally needed to be healthy and to thrive.

I had always known that food can either be the most powerful source of healing or the slowest form of poison. My problem was I had placed my nutritional ladder up against the wrong wall. I was systematically following a dietary lifestyle that was not working for my cellular physiology, my mental wellbeing, my hormones or my energy. Step by step, I was climbing the ladder to an increasingly tired body and undernourished brain.

I started to understand the impact sugar was having on my brain, where the continuous glucose load being dumped into the bloodstream was sending the feel-good chemical dopamine soaring, in the same way that alcohol and drugs do. Over time, the drive to devour sugar increases in order to meet the high levels of dopamine the brain has come to expect, essentially demanding more, distracting you from a narrative other than … I want more sugar, NOW!

As hunter-gatherers, we are designed to seek out sweet, seasonal berries, perfecting our foraging skills by forming strong memories of taste, smell and sensory experiences, forging this relationship of our love for the sweet stuff through a heady dose of a 'this feels wonderful' dopamine hit.

These strong cues are carved out in the brain, in preparation for the next season of sweet berries as you roam the land in search of food. However, this is not how our modern food environment works. At odds with the environment of scarcity, we don't have to forage, roam and remember, instead we find ourselves deliberating in aisle nine as to whether we should really be adding glazed doughnuts to the trolley as our brain enthusiastically reminds us of just how good they're going to taste.

These powerful drivers in the brain inhibit your executive control; you're a very intelligent, fully grown adult who knows a six-pack of iced buns spells trouble, but this part of your brain becomes overridden by the motivation and 'pay attention' centres that are lighting up as you walk past the rows and rows of triggers calling to you and reminding you to not worry about that sensible stuff, you need to eat me, now! In that moment, our inhibitory control becomes distinctly inhibited!

There is a science to navigating eating in the modern world that involves biology as well as psychology, and the two go hand in hand. Have you ever wondered why sometimes you eat and just can't feel satisfied, how despite making a pact to change, you find yourself back in your old habits the very next day? We must work with our physiology as well as understand the impact that our emotions and brain chemistry have on the success of a healthy relationship with food in order to create better health and lasting change.

Fall in Love with Taking Care of Yourself

'Do the best you can until you know better. Then when you know better, do better.'

— MAYA ANGELOU

For me, shame reared its ugly head regularly. If you've ever overeaten, tried to diet, binge-eaten or struggled with self-control, you'll know exactly how shame seeps into every cell of your body, driving low self-worth and feelings of hopelessness.

It was only when I really began to understand the impact that food was having on my brain chemistry – volatile blood sugars driving the desire for more, creating dysregulation in hunger and satiety hormones and helping to stomp down emotions I was afraid to feel – that I could see the destructive pathway I had been on. The food choices I was making were leaving me feeling dead long before they would actually kill me.

I decided, after the thousandth time of 'trying to give up sugar' and get healthy, that rather than feel shameful and worthless, I would look for an opportunity to learn from what my body was telling me. I was clearly hooked on the sweet stuff, but why?

I had wired my brain to desire sugar in a very powerful way, which was driving my food choices, making me feel increasingly tired and disrupting both my sex and hunger hormones. Shame was hindering my progress; this soul-eating emotion was the first thing I had to lose. Without ditching the shame, I knew the sugar would find its way back to me, like a long-lost friend.

I needed a plan, a plan that would work when I felt good, motivated and inspired, but also one that would catch me before I fell, a plan that would stop me running back to the clutches of sugar when life got hard and my emotions were feeling fraught. I knew that the battle began first in my head, between what I knew was the right path to take, versus the strong desire to just eat what I wanted.

'These pains you feel are messages, listen to them.'

— RUMI

Connection is the best protection against relapsing into a habit you are trying to break. Re-establishing the connection with yourself, hearing the hurt that may have driven your decisions to drown out pain with food, wine or other state-changing behaviours. Acknowledging the pain, trauma and emotions that have been carried for years that must now be let go of in order to move forward and create a peaceful relationship with food – one that doesn't drive hurt, pain and frustration but instead cultivates enjoyment, delight and nourishment. It should allow you to fall in love with taking care of yourself.

This pathway takes planning, preparation and protection from the challenges of living in a food environment that can trigger you to fall back into old ways at the sniff of a doughnut or the sight of a custard cream. Planning is key, because planning enables you to make a decision about something and prepare in advance, so you know what you will have in your cupboards and your fridge. Planning is imperative because it takes the negotiation out of whether to have the chocolate bar calling from the kitchen, because when you know it's in there, you know it's there, and it calls upon the part of your brain that sees you heading to eat it even when you know you don't want to. Our memories of just how good these foods taste are hardwired into our procedural memory, a subconscious part of our brain that functions below our consciousness and makes it incredibly challenging to inhibit!

Our brains are very smart at getting what they want, so we need to outsmart our brains. This takes a little planning, some home truths and some preparation.

Overwhelm can easily set in when we are planning a new, healthier way of eating. This overwhelm can lead to self-sabotage. I know some of you are nodding your heads right now; hands up, come on, hands up who has been there? Plan the meals for the week but focus your attention on a day-by-day basis. This will give you the strength to focus your attention just on today. When the negotiations in your head begin – the strong desire telling you to 'eat the cream doughnut' – do not fight it; simply acknowledge the desire, staying calm, and state to yourself in your head: I'm not eating that today, not today.

Focus on one day at a time. These individual days soon add up and you will find yourself a week in, a month in and your desire for sugar, the cravings, the clutch of the sweet stuff is loosening. You haven't battled yourself, you've not given energy to the struggle, instead you have remained calm and focused on the day-to-day, which lowers stress and allows you to make better decisions, which ultimately results in lasting change.

Your Health Destiny

Having been a people-pleaser for most of my life, I felt selfish if I considered my own needs before those of my children, husband, work, friends and family. However, in behaving in this way, the message I was inadvertently giving myself was that I wasn't good enough, I wasn't worthy, and that message was driven deeper every time I blurred boundaries that I should have been setting in place. When I stopped this destructive behaviour and recognised that I had to serve myself first, I realised it put me in the best position to support those I love, to be the best mother, wife, friend, sister. I was enough … and so are you. Set clear boundaries and reinforce the love you have for yourself by keeping to them.

I took my health into my own hands, taking responsibility for where it was, acknowledging the mess I'd made for my body to clean up. But I didn't linger there; I felt acceptance and excitement about a new pathway, one that would lead me to health, happiness and hormonal balance – one that has led me to here, to you.

Nine years on and my life is considerably different. My body is stronger, my relationship with food healthier and my hunger is under control. I have more capacity for focus, for learning, for retaining information, as well as more clarity of thought. Yes, I have bad days just like everyone else, but I don't allow myself to stay there; my outlook on life is different because my brain responds differently now. It has the nutrients it needs to thrive. It lights up, brimming with ideas, trillions of neurons firing and communicating at unthinkable speed and connectivity. Life now vibrates in a full spectrum of colour, my senses find beauty in the simplest of scenarios – trees waving cheerfully in the sea breeze, the distinctively delicious smell of mint leaves in my kitchen, the clasping warmth of my children's hands as we cross the road, the tender kiss of my husband before bed, the first bite of warm wholesome carrot and apple muffin (yes, the recipe is in here, see page 224). My brain now seeks out possibility in the difficult and serves to find ways to challenge yet nurture growth. Emotions brim at the edge of my heart but now anger, frustration and hurt are replaced by peace, love and kindness. The key to creating the seemingly impossible? A fully nourished brain and body, the true foundation of our ultimate health and wellbeing.

My diet and lifestyle look very different to those of nine years ago. Having spent years researching and understanding the science of our primal health, cellular and physiological needs, I made steady and lasting changes. I quickly noticed improvements. My body responded for the first time in a long while in the way I had hoped, losing weight, gaining energy and feeling myself again. The more I learned, the more changes I made. I researched what it really meant to be healthy. I studied for a Masters in Nutrition, Physical Activity and Public Health, deepening my knowledge and scientific grounding in a subject I had now become completely immersed in.

And now over to you … You are the gatekeeper, you are the creator of your masterpiece. You are in control of your own health destiny. Wherever you are with your health right now, the struggles you are having, it's time for acceptance and to make peace as you gear yourself up for a new ride, a new journey of exploration and adventure. Our ability to draw a line under the past and begin afresh, erasing old habits and moving forward with new eyes, new energy and new choices, is the one thing we all have in common. Our relentlessly forgiving bodies will respond to this and eagerly agree to it.

It is my hope that when you begin to understand how mind-blowingly brilliant you are, you will begin to see yourself as just that. Eating well will become a form of self-respect, a daily display of self-love.

The domino effect of sugar cravings, overeating, constant hunger, hormonal imbalances, stubborn weight, tiredness and low mood are all linked in a slippery slope that starts with what we eat and how we fuel our hungry brain! A fully nourished brain and body, freedom from cravings, hormonal balance and vibrant energy are the true foundation of health and wellbeing. The principles of how to eat to satisfy hunger, hormonal balance and happiness will be covered in this book, offering empowering and easy-to-implement solutions.

Let's begin by getting to know ourselves a little better – starting with our hormones.

Two

Meet Your Hormones

As young girls our sex hormones remain fairly quiet until oestrogen bursts onto the scene at puberty, making her presence known. This first flurry into womanhood sees our body shapes change as oestrogen starts directing the show, instructing fat to be laid down on the thighs, hips and breasts, carving out our womanly curves.

From oestrogen's first big entrance, it's clear that this hormone is in charge; left unchecked, oestrogen becomes overbearing and dominant. All over-excitable friends need a calming side-kick, and in this case that calming influence of oestrogen's wild ways is progesterone.

In the party of life, oestrogen is at centre stage, jumping on the tables and letting loose. Oestrogen influences everyone in her presence and is loved by all … in the right doses – but too much and the party gets out of hand. Progesterone is the party guest your teenage self would have hated but your parents would have loved – turning down the music a little, putting coasters under the glasses, encouraging oestrogen down off the table. Progesterone brings calm, keeps oestrogen in check and helps reduce tension. Progesterone is the peacekeeper.

Understanding the relationship between oestrogen and progesterone is important. As we navigate through our female lives, the delicate dance between these two vital sex hormones can fall out of balance, leaving oestrogen to exert her dominance and progesterone to be elbowed off the scene. This results in many of the signs and symptoms of hormonal imbalances that we have become accustomed to – heavy periods, painful cramping, PMS, stubborn weight gain, anxiety, sleeplessness. All of these can be driven by the absence or presence of key sex hormones and their changing ratio. Understanding the roles that these hormones play, what constitutes a 'normal' menstrual cycle and why certain symptoms arise during our monthly cycle, allows us to consciously choose dietary and lifestyle habits that support the balance of our sex hormones.

The Sex Hormones

Our sex hormones do what they say on the tin: they support our reproductive needs. However, alongside baby-making, there is a whole spectrum of jobs that Mother Nature considers essential for successful reproduction – from our mood and sociability, to sex drive, sexual characteristics and sexual behaviour – before we even get to fertility. Our sex-hormone balance impacts many aspects of our physiology and behaviour – they are powerful hormones!

As women, our monthly cycle can be a real insight into the balance – or imbalance – of our sex hormones. Having normalised many of the symptoms we experience, from heavy periods, irregular periods, PMS, painful periods, anxiety and weight gain, we may have lost sight of what's normal and what is not when it comes to our menstrual cycle.

OESTROGEN

Crucial for growth and development, oestrogen generally drives the 'building' of tissues such as the thickening of the womb lining in preparation for pregnancy, the building of strong bones and of collagen – an important protein that brings structural integrity to the skin and other tissues of the body. Oestrogen has many other roles, too, such as preserving bone health and preventing osteoporosis, as well as providing cardioprotective and neuroprotective support.

Oestrogen has broader implications that can help us understand our changing body, because the levels of this important hormone increase and decrease over our female lifetime. Oestrogen directs where fat is stored on the body, encouraging fat deposition on the hips, thighs and breast. Oestrogen also plays a role in supporting insulin to usher blood sugars into the cells (more on the importance of this later!). Oestrogen also impacts our appetite. In the days leading up to our period, we can feel hungrier as oestrogen levels lower, while oestrogen levels peak just prior to ovulation, a time when we generally feel less hungry.

The peaks and troughs of our oestrogen levels across the monthly cycle reflect the role that this hormone plays in our mood, energy levels and sex drive. When oestrogen levels are low on the first day of menstruation, our mood is reflective of this, and we are more prone to anxiety, feeling introverted and seeking out comforting foods, rest and light forms of exercise.

As oestrogen starts to rise in the follicular phase, we begin to feel brighter, more sociable and energised. As oestrogen reaches peak levels, ovulation is stimulated alongside a peak in testosterone. Motivation, sex drive and competitiveness are all at their optimum levels at this time. At ovulation there is a drop in oestrogen, followed by a gradual increase, but it is progesterone that really peaks in this luteal phase, increasing feelings of calm and inner peace.

PROGESTERONE

Progesterone is a pro-pregnancy hormone, which helps to maintain a viable pregnancy and support the developing embryo. Progesterone is produced in large amounts following ovulation in the luteal phase of the menstrual cycle. If pregnancy doesn't occur, progesterone levels quickly fall and the endometrial lining breaks down and triggers a menstrual bleed and the first day of your period. Progesterone, in essence, helps to keep the endometrial lining in place.

Progesterone is your 'keep calm and carry on' hormone, having a positive impact on GABA (gamma aminobutyric acid), a calming neurotransmitter that soothes and quietens an over-anxious brain. Progesterone stimulates GABA, which tells your brain to quit the jibba jabba and overthinking, allowing for relaxation, calm and a good night's sleep.

Go with the Flow

What does hormonal balance look and feel like? A good starting place for checking in with our hormones is our monthly cycle; this can offer great insight into the delicate balance between oestrogen and progesterone, offering understanding of symptoms that can accompany oestrogen dominance, low progesterone or low oestrogen and why these imbalances occur. It is always important to check with your doctor if you have any symptoms of concern, such as vaginal bleeding that is unusual for you – including bleeding during or after sex, bleeding between periods, pain during sex or any concerns with vaginal discharge.

What 'normal' looks like for you specifically does depend on your age, lifestyle, past medical history and genetics. There is no real average or 'normal' as we are all so unique, however, certain parameters can guide us in understanding what is considered a healthy 'normal' menstrual cycle. Tracking our cycle in our twenties and thirties can be very helpful, then from our forties onwards we enter a new phase of hormonal change, the perimenopause. At this time, we can really start to notice changes during our cycle – including our mood, weight changes, sleep disturbance, anxiety levels, as well as changes to our cycle – heaviness, blood colour, flow and cycle length. However, it is never too late to start understanding and tracking your menstrual cycle!

WHAT ARE THE INDICATIONS THAT OUR HORMONES ARE BALANCED?

The more we understand what a healthy cycle looks and feels like, the easier it is to make the necessary shifts to our diet and lifestyle to support our hormonal health. In this way, hormonal changes through our female lifespan become easier to spot, understand and support.

So what are the signs we should be looking out for?

Length of cycle

The textbook length of a menstrual cycle is twenty-eight days. However, women can have a longer or shorter cycle and still have hormonal balance. The average menstrual length is twenty-nine days, but a healthy cycle can range from twenty-five to thirty-five days.

Cycle length is determined by the length of the follicular phase – the first half of the menstrual cycle. Oestrogen has to reach a certain level in order for ovulation to occur and for the second half of the menstrual cycle, the luteal phase, to progress. When oestrogen levels are high, shorter cycles with heavier bleeds can result. When cycles are longer, it can be due to lower levels of oestrogen taking longer to reach the necessary threshold for ovulation to occur. The correct amount of oestrogen and progesterone is necessary in order to determine the length of cycle and length of the menstrual bleed.

The long and short of it

How long we bleed for can give us great insight into the balance of our hormones. Bleed length and heaviness are also important considerations in understanding the nutrient levels that may alter when we have consistently long and heavy periods. Magnesium and iron levels may lower, leaving us vulnerable to anaemia and the symptoms of subclinical magnesium deficiency – anxiety, poor sleep, migraines, muscle tension and cramping, constipation and low energy (more on this in Chapter Five).

The average menstrual bleed is between three and seven days in length. Adequate levels of oestrogen are necessary to build up the uterine lining and sufficient levels of progesterone are required to slow the build-up of the lining. This perfect balance of build-up and slow down between oestrogen and progesterone results in a period of three to seven days in length, one that isn't too heavy or too light. A day or two prior to your menstrual bleed, you may experience some darker-coloured brown spotting, which is normal and indicative of old blood left over from your last period. Three days or more of spotting before your period can indicate that progesterone levels are low or falling, as can happen during the early stages of perimenopause. When progesterone levels become low, spotting can occur as progesterone is unable to adequately do its job and keep the uterine lining in place. Flooding of blood in the first few days of your period is also a sign of low progesterone, again because the absence of adequate levels of progesterone is preventing the uterine lining being held in place. Low progesterone can also lead to issues with fertility and miscarriage, fatigue and low libido.

Through thick and thin

The colour and consistency of our menstrual blood can give us a snapshot of the balance of our sex hormones. Menstrual blood is a mixture of red blood cells, vaginal fluid and endometrial tissue lining. Blood colour varies from fire-engine red to pink or dark brown. Darker brown often indicates slower-moving blood, which can be due to a flexed uterus slowing the passage and flow of the blood. Lighter, watery blood can be due to lower levels of oestrogen causing insufficient building of the uterine lining, or low levels of iron. The consistency should flow easily. Thick, sticky blood with large numbers of clots can indicate higher levels of oestrogen and low progesterone. Some clotting is normal, however, clots over an inch in size could indicate oestrogen dominance.

Volume

Determining the amount of blood loss during our monthly cycles can be a little challenging, for obvious reasons. However, we can get a fairly good idea as to the volume of blood loss by the amount of period protection we are using and how regularly we are having to change to measure that protection. The amount of blood loss during a healthy monthly bleed is 30–60ml. One regular pad or tampon holds approximately 5ml of blood, so for an average period we would be looking at using six to ten tampons or pads; 80ml per cycle would be considered heavy.

Periods can be particularly heavy for the first few days, with flooding and doubling up of period protection necessary. This is indicative of low progesterone and oestrogen dominance. Pay attention to how many pads or tampons you are going through per cycle – or the volume of blood in your menstrual cup – how regularly you are having to replace your protection and the pattern of blood loss; for instance, if it is very heavy in the first few days or throughout your bleed.

A light period would be considered 25ml of blood loss or less and can indicate low oestrogen, particularly if accompanied by longer-length cycles and watery, thin period blood. However, don't forget we are ALL different and these figures are simply an indication, a guide on understanding your hormones a little better!

Common Hormonal Imbalances

Our hormonal lifecycle is influenced by environmental factors such as emotional stress, stimulants and hormone-disrupting chemicals called endocrine disruptors, as well as our diet and nutritional deficiencies, blood sugars and insulin sensitivity, gut health, liver function, exercise and sleep. We are at risk of hormonal imbalances at any stage of our female lifespan, however, various stages of our female life offer different challenges and risks of hormonal imbalances.

PUBERTY ▶

MENOPAUSE ▶

High oestrogen
Low progesterone
—
Hormones are fluctuating, periods can be heavy until progesterone establishes itself on the scene. Prone to anxiety, poor sleep, fatigue, easy bruising, PMS and low mood. Also prone to low iron and magnesium levels if periods are heavy.

Low oestrogen
Low progesterone
—
Insulin resistance, poor metabolic health and chronic stress can exacerbate and prolong the adaption of the brain to lower levels of oestrogen and progesterone. Prone to brain fog, memory issues, hot flushes, prolonged hunger, weight gain, low mood, depression, insomnia and fatigue.

High oestrogen
Low progesterone
—
Following years of chronic stress and 'doing too much for too long', progesterone levels tend to be low and oestrogen high. Prone to heavy periods, fatigue, anxiety, insomnia, weight gain, skin issues, increased allergies, digestive issues and low mood.

Balanced oestrogen
Balanced progesterone
—
Oestrogen dominance and PCOS can be common at this stage of life. Having a baby settles hormones in some women, in others it leads to hormonal disruption. Hormones are heavily influenced by diet, lifestyle and stress. Prone to anxiety, insomnia, low mood and fertility issues.

▶ **TWENTIES AND THIRTIES**

▶ **PERIMENOPAUSE**

PUBERTY AND TEENS

The transition from childhood into adulthood offers a rude awakening to the world of hormones and their power and influence over our body shape, emotions and behaviour. Teenage girls and young women tend to have irregular cycles, with more frequent or heavier bleeding as the two sex hormones become synchronised in their newfound roles. Initially, lower levels of progesterone in relation to oestrogen can result in heavier, painful periods, erratic cycles, high levels of irritability and increased levels of anxiety. As progesterone finds her footing, balancing out the heavy presence of oestrogen, periods can settle down in late teenage years and as women enter their twenties.

TWENTIES AND THIRTIES

Life really begins to get interesting in these two decades; the early twenties can see a change in living arrangements and independent dietary choices as we fly the nest. Free to make all those decisions yourself – eating what you want, when you want. Alcohol can weave its way into the picture during your late teens and twenties, with a heavy presence for many through to your thirties as we attempt to cope with the demands of family life, work life, social life and life in general!

Job changes, baby-making, multiple stressors; life in our twenties and thirties can see our teenage hormones settle quite nicely, or flip-flop into dysfunction, creating fertility issues, Polycystic Ovary Syndrome (PCOS), problematic skin, PMS, heavy bleeding topped off with exhaustion and anxiety. Layering hormonal disturbances on top of an already hectic and challenging life leads to food and lifestyle choices becoming a coping mechanism that often further exacerbates our imbalanced female sex hormones.

Pregnancy can certainly impact the sex hormones – and for some in a beneficial way, leading to improved regularity and flow of periods and the accompanying symptoms. For others, pregnancy can trigger hormonal imbalances as the challenges of motherhood, pressures of modern life, dietary disruption, sleep disturbance and emotional stress all add to the rollercoaster ride that sees you exhausted and frustrated with your weight, mood and manic hormones.

With so many contributing factors impacting hormones in these two decades, no two experiences are ever the same for women. However, one thing that is becoming increasingly evident is that the decades leading up to our forties have a cumulative impact on the transition from perimenopause to menopause. Remember, it is never too early or late to focus on optimising hormonal health!

The reality for many women is that as we reach thirty-five years of age our hormonal profile starts to change. This may surprise you, as it seems young to be experiencing hormonal shifts, however, it is at this age that we begin to see levels of key hormones lower, and this can impact our weight, metabolic rate, muscle mass and mood. From thirty-five onwards, what and when we eat, as well as our lifestyle choices, become increasingly influential on our weight status, more than they were in years gone by. We will take a closer look at the important fat-storing and metabolism-impacting actions of hormones in Chapter Three.

Changes to our sex hormone profile really kick in as we approach our late thirties and they fully establish their presence in our forties, but before we look at this key period in our female hormonal lives – perimenopause – let's look at some common hormonal imbalances that women experience from their teenage years through to perimenopause.

Oestrogen Dominance

Oestrogen dominance is very common in women of pre-menopausal age, so much so that it has almost become synonymous with modern life. It is a powerful and dominant hormone that requires the delicate balance and presence of progesterone in order to blunt its impact on many of the tissues in the body. Think of oestrogen as your front lawn, growing thick and rapidly; it needs progesterone, the lawnmower, to keep it in check. When progesterone is low, oestrogen dominates and drives the symptoms that have become normalised as 'period problems' and that are often accepted as part of being a woman: heavy periods, short cycles, PMS, irritability, anxiety, fibrocystic breasts, water retention, migraines, fibroids and endometriosis.

Maintaining a balance between the two main female sex hormones of oestrogen and progesterone therefore has major beneficial implications on our mood, weight, body shape, bone health, heart health and menstrual cycle. Oestrogen levels naturally shift over the menstrual cycle, increasing from ten to a hundred-fold over a twenty-eight-day period and this hormone exerts its effects wide and far across the body, with a high proportion of oestrogen receptors found in the brain, all musculoskeletal tissue, including bone, muscle, tendons and ligaments, as well as the central nervous system and cardiovascular system.

What drives this imbalance of oestrogen and progesterone?

Hormonal disruptors come in all shapes and sizes in our modern-day lives. From what we think to the foods we eat, the minute-by-minute impact of these foods, thoughts and our environment on our hormonal balance is continuous. Understanding the impact of what we eat, in particular, and its ability to influence our hormones, offers us a much deeper level of knowledge and control over our hormonal health and overall wellbeing. In Chapter Three, we will explore the key hormone that is disrupting dietary and lifestyle behaviours and how we can adapt our diet to eat foods that promote hormonal balance, optimal weight, health and happiness.

Polycystic Ovary Syndrome

PCOS is the most common cause of infertility in women. A complex syndrome and not always easy to diagnose, it is mostly associated with resistant weight, cravings, hunger and insulin resistance. High levels of insulin not only drive fat storage and essentially block attempts at weight loss, but are also at the heart of PCOS.

As previously discussed, high levels of oestrogen are needed to trigger ovulation, and in the absence of a peak in oestrogen, ovulation is absent, leading to fertility issues. All oestrogen originates as testosterone, with the ovaries converting testosterone into oestrogen via an important enzyme called aromatase. Insulin blocks the activity of this enzyme, leading to high levels of testosterone and low levels of oestrogen. The higher levels of testosterone cause symptoms typically associated with PCOS, such as increased facial hair, hair loss at the crown of the head, skin breakouts, longer menstrual cycles, a deeper voice and even aggressive tendencies.

Managing insulin resistance, blood sugars and what and when we eat are at the centre of addressing this hormonal imbalance. Whether we are dominant in testosterone or oestrogen, optimising blood sugars and insulin sensitivity and providing the nutrients needed for hormone building and stress reduction are all key components of a sustainable hormone-balancing diet and lifestyle.

PERIMENOPAUSE ... *A TIME OF TRANSITION*

'Life is a series of natural and spontaneous changes. Don't resist them – that only creates sorrow. Let reality be reality. Let things flow naturally forward in whatever way they like.'

— LAO TZU

In my younger years I believed that menopause was a switch that came along and turned off our fertility as we entered our fifties, an 'event' more than a transitory period. After some major 'aha' moments, I realised that waving adios to our fertile years is much less a swift departure of progesterone and oestrogen, but more a gradual easing out of these hormones. Much like teenagers moving out of the family home, oestrogen and progesterone make their departure gradually – and in the case of oestrogen, rather erratically!

Migraines, heavy bleeding, painful periods, insomnia, breast tenderness, skin issues; for many women, perimenopause can feel like the return of puberty. From the age of forty years old, there is a definite shift in our hormonal landscape. This key period in our female lives sees us gradually transition from our fertile years to a time of reproductive retirement. This period, which can last between eight and ten years, is called perimenopause and is split into two distinct phases defined by what is happening to oestrogen and progesterone during those times.

The early stages of perimenopause see progesterone levels gradually and steadily decline in a predictable manner. Oestrogen levels, on the other hand, are far more erratic, and with the decline of progesterone, the symptoms of oestrogen dominance can set in.

Stage one perimenopause ... the second puberty

Oestrogen dominance in our forties can feel wildly frustrating. The feelings of increased anxiety, the heavy painful periods, headaches, skin changes, irrational behaviour, poor sleep, weight gain and changing body shape are direct results of lowering progesterone levels, erratic oestrogen and a shift in our metabolic hormones (more on this in Chapter Three).

Perimenopause becomes a barometer of our health, shining a spotlight on underlying, long-standing hormonal imbalances that have accumulated from our twenties, thirties and forties. Doing too much for too long leads to emotional and physical exhaustion, poor dietary habits, poor gut health, blood sugar issues and detrimental lifestyle habits, and these all add up and take centre stage during perimenopause, demanding attention at a time when you may feel least equipped and able to deal with it.

Understanding the impact that our day-to-day choices have, at all ages and stages of our female lives, on our hormones and our female physiology is key in preparing mentally and physically for perimenopause and beyond.

Changes associated with early perimenopause

As ovulation starts to slow down from our mid-thirties onwards, progesterone levels slowly decline, leaving oestrogen to exert its dominance on the various tissues of the body, particularly the brain. The brain has one of the highest densities of oestrogen receptors. Mood changes, headaches, irrational and erratic behaviour can all accompany this time of change. As progesterone is our 'keep calm and carry on' hormone, the departure of this soothing hormone can hit our mood and sleep hard at this time. Insomnia and sleep deprivation worsen the symptoms of perimenopause, further disrupting blood sugar stability, increasing hunger hormones, lowering satiety hormones and driving over-eating.

Testosterone is often thought of as a male sex hormone, however, women actually have more testosterone than circulating oestrogen. Testosterone levels need to be 'just right' for us ladies; too much and we can experience the symptoms of PCOS, too little impacts our muscle building, metabolism and motivation. Men have levels of testosterone that are ten times higher than those of women, giving them a 'testosterone advantage' when it comes to losing weight. Our testosterone levels decline during perimenopause, which can lead to a lower sex drive, increased fatigue, lower confidence and motivation.

Stage two perimenopause

The second phase of perimenopause sees oestrogen levels leave the dominant state and begin to decline. Your periods reflect this by becoming lighter, with more spotting and longer-length cycles. This decline in oestrogen, coupled with low progesterone, brings new challenges, commonly experienced as low mood, depression, brain fog and memory issues, hot flushes, night sweats, heart palpitations, energy dips, fatigue, loss of libido and internal dryness.

While oestrogen is well known as a sex hormone, it also plays important roles in metabolic health, enhancing insulin sensitivity and reducing the likelihood of type 2 diabetes. As oestrogen levels decline, there is an increased tendency to store weight around the belly.

Oestrogen helps insulin to usher glucose from the blood into the cells, providing fuel for energy. As oestrogen levels lower, less glucose is available to areas of the brain that need it for fuel. This can be destabilising to your brain and nervous system. Areas of the brain responsible for temperature control, hunger, memory, fear and focus receive less fuel as oestrogen levels lower, leaving those areas of the brain under-fuelled. This is further exacerbated by a state called insulin resistance (see page 47), which can worsen and prolong the symptoms of perimenopause and menopause.

Women are two to four times more likely to suffer major depressive episodes during perimenopause or in early and post-menopause, according to the Study of Women's Health Across the Nation (SWAN). Building a healthy, resilient brain and nervous system is key for optimising hormonal balance and reducing the occurrence of depressive episodes.

Optimising insulin sensitivity and stabilising blood sugars is a key component of hormonal balance. Eating to optimise insulin sensitivity, with a nutrient-dense diet packed with magnesium, B vitamins, protein, fibre and some healthy fats, will help you feel fuller for longer, stabilise your blood sugars, optimise your metabolic hormones and help to balance your sex hormones.

MENOPAUSE

After navigating the highs and lows of perimenopause, the menopause arrives, officially defined as twelve months following your last period at the average age of fifty-one. Oestrogen levels have now tapered down from the second stage of perimenopause and we face new and ongoing challenges. However, just as with perimenopause, understanding and anticipating these challenges allows us to plan for and protect ourselves.

Our inherently wise female body responds to low levels of oestrogen by increasing oestrogen receptor numbers and sensitivity. Oestrogen, once made by the ovaries, is now made from a precursor compound called DHEA, which is produced within the adrenal glands. The adrenals are situated above the kidneys and are responsible for making our stress hormones. Looking after our adrenals in the years and decades leading up to menopause ensures the shift from ovarian production of oestrogen to the adrenal glands is a smooth transition.

Oestrogen production, previously occurring in the ovaries, now happens within the cells of the brain, bones, muscle, liver and heart. Testosterone, made from DHEA, is converted to oestrogen via the enzyme aromatase. The activity of aromatase increases during menopause, another way of ensuring we have enough oestrogen. Accurately gauging oestrogen levels now becomes challenging since oestrogen production happens within the cells of the various tissues and is not circulating in the blood in the same way as pre-menopause.

Oestrogen exists in three main forms: oestriol, produced during pregnancy, oestradiol, which is dominant during pre-menopausal years, and oestrone, produced following menopause. Body fat is also a source of oestrone production, with too much body fat increasing the risk of breast cancer, endometrial cancer and abnormal bleeding. Body weight can be an issue for many women, particularly post-menopausally, which can see our metabolic rate drop by 15 per cent with an increased risk of insulin resistance. The main influencers of metabolic rate and how to shift stubborn body weight will be covered in Chapter Three.

Nature's Plan

We are not designed to suffer; nature has a plan. We are hardwired for reproduction and all that happens within our monthly cycle of hormonal change is exquisitely designed to optimise our chances of conceiving and carrying that baby to full term. We suffer when our physiology cannot adapt fast enough to our changing environment; when our modern diet and lifestyle collide with the natural ebbs and flows of our hormonal system, we end up fighting a losing battle.

Stop fighting and start embracing

Often in life we end up feeling like we are battling ourselves, willing ourselves to be stronger, better, more disciplined, more successful, younger, slimmer. Embracing our female physiology means understanding how best to work with our body, in a modern world that is often at odds with our nutritional and physiological needs.

We live in a time when we understand more than ever about human science and yet so many women suffer during this life-changing transition. As I write this book in my early forties many of my female friends speak of their struggles, lack of knowledge or preparation during this important transitional phase of perimenopause. What's more frustrating is the disempowering way in which menopause is spoken about. The way we view this time of change is something that many women seem to fear, anticipating preconceived ideas perpetuated by a mainstream narrative.

Change we don't want is harder to embrace than change we choose, such as starting a new job or moving house. Inevitable change can leave us feeling vulnerable and out of control. We must begin by understanding the powerful influence we have during this time of hormonal change, in order to regain confidence and mastery over our bodies.

Let's take a look at the main hormonal disruptors and how we can begin to build a diet and lifestyle that supports our hormones, health and happiness.

Three

The Big Disruptors

Now we have a much better understanding of how our sex hormones influence every facet of our females lives, what we really want to do is get down to the crux of this book: what is disrupting our hormones, interrupting great sleep, worsening anxiety, causing stubborn weight gain and *what do we do about it*?

Recreating hormonal harmony is rarely about addressing one individual food or habit; we must identify all our dietary and lifestyle practices that cause disruption and make adjustments, step-by-step, to bring about balance and lasting change. For this book, I have taken decades of learning and understanding of complex concepts and broken them down into five simple, easy-to-apply core principles. While we are all individuals with various needs, genetic differences and biological variances, these principles can be applied to most of us in order to optimise energy, metabolic flexibility, hormonal health and mental wellbeing. They are based upon the laws of nature, our physiological systems and how our health spirals down when we go against those laws, but also on how we can flourish when we work with our female physiology.

Before we delve into the five core principles, first we will take a walk through the common, everyday practices that we undertake that are undermining our best efforts to lose weight, gain energy and balance. What are we doing on a daily basis that is undoing all those hours in the gym? All the discipline you might be putting into your diet without seeing the results? Your loyal and faithful servant, your body, is ready and waiting to respond to change. Are you ready?

The Lowdown on Insulin

Insulin resistance worsens and prolongs the symptoms of perimenopause and the menopause. You may or may not have heard of insulin resistance, however, we are going to do a little biology 101 here because insulin and insulin resistance play a BIG part in our weight, mood, memory, hunger, energy, fertility, inflammation and long-term health. Basically it's key in understanding what has gone awry and, most importantly, how we fix it!

What is insulin and why should I care?!

Insulin is a hormone that has *great* influence over whether we burn or store fat. Insulin wants the body to store energy, it is the Martin Lewis of the endocrine world – super efficient at energy saving and fat-storing, piling it onto our hips, butt and belly for a rainy day. Why burn fat when you can store it?! While Martin's fat-storing instructions would have been essential for our hunter-gatherer ancestors when food was scarce and we were uncertain when our next bush full of berries or wild bison would be available, our food environment and the type of food we eat are now vastly different from those of our caveman predecessors. When super-saver Martin is continuously on the scene, we never get to access that rainy day stored fund of fat to burn.

Insulin is a hormone produced by the pancreas that we simply cannot survive without, however the right amount of insulin is key – not too much, not too little. When we eat, our blood sugar level rises, how much depends on *what* we eat. The rise in blood sugar triggers insulin to come along and usher the sugars from our blood into our cells for fuel. This system works well when glucose is present, as it gets shunted into the cells by insulin to use for fuel. When glucose is absent, though, glucagon, an opposing hormone to insulin (think Martin Lewis's nemesis, burn ALL the fat stores, spend, spend, spend!), signals for fat to be released and burned for energy. When there are excessive amounts of glucose that aren't being burned for fuel (for example, if we eat more than the body is burning), the excess glucose is converted by the liver into fat. Can we change how much energy we burn (our metabolic rate)? Why, yes, we can! More on that later.

The ability to burn both glucose and fat essentially make us dual-fuel burners, burning sugar for fuel when it's available or fat from our body when it's not. However, we rarely give our body the opportunity to access the fat reserves because of our eating habits – what we eat and when we eat mean our glucose and insulin levels rarely lower to the point of welcoming glucagon to the stage to start directing fat-burning.

Our dual-fuel-burning status means we can survive during times of scarcity, because our physiological needs are essentially hardwired to provide us with the greatest odds of survival. Our philosophising, what-is-the-meaning-of-life brains might jeer at the thought that our life merely comes down to passing on our genetic material, but there's no arguing with your DNA. So how does this seemingly simple and effective system end up going so wrong?!

Insulin resistance

Insulin resistance will hamper your *best* attempts to lose weight and burn fat. Years of high-sugar eating, stress and inflammation all contribute to this very modern problem called insulin resistance. Cells become deaf to the demands of insulin to 'take in more glucose', and essentially insulin stops functioning as it should. Blood sugars begin to rise and yet more insulin has to be produced by the pancreas in an attempt to mop up ever-rising levels of blood sugars. As insulin resistance kicks in, less glucose is able to enter the cells, leaving you under-fuelled, hungry and tired, but with higher blood sugar levels that are now being converted into body and liver fat. Insulin levels also rise, blocking fat burning. Current thinking is that insulin resistance rather than overeating drives obesity.

How do I know if I have insulin resistance?

If you are a little overweight and have consistently high blood pressure, it is likely you have a degree of insulin resistance. The skin can also be a good indicator of insulin resistance; skin tags near the armpits, neck and groin and dark patches of discoloured skin, a condition called acanthosis nigricans, can also indicate insulin resistance. Strong sugar cravings and skin breakouts are other clues that you may have insulin resistance.

What causes insulin resistance?

Chronically elevated levels of blood sugars eventually lead to chronically elevated levels of insulin. Living a low-insulin lifestyle is the first habit of hormonal balance, and this is easier than you might think. Diet plays a part, as we have just discovered, spiking our blood sugars and leading to spikes in our insulin, but there are other considerations outside of diet that drive insulin levels up, up and away …

What You Eat and
When You Eat it

What you eat impacts your hormones. Truth bomb number one: food is not just fuel, food talks to your hormones and this little chat ends up directing you to gain weight, lose weight, lose sleep, feel great, feel terrible … You name it, our hormones are involved and our hormones are hugely influenced by the food we eat.

FAT FOR FUEL

Our body will choose to burn fat for fuel when glucose is not an option. In other words, we turn to this incredible reserve of fuel we are carrying around with us, conveniently stored on our butts and hips, ready to burn and give us the energy we need to get going for the day.

However – and here is the kicker – if we have a continuous presence of glucose and insulin, that reserve of fat stays decidedly put. Insulin will keep attempting to push more and more glucose into the cells, with any excess being converted into fat and stored as fuel to use later.

THE HUNGRY BRAIN

Our brains are hungry beasts. They demand a high level of fuel … all the time. Muscles are also high up on the energy-demanding scale. When we eat food with a high carbohydrate load this is efficiently broken down into a usable source of fuel for our body: glucose. The glucose from our panini, pasta, porridge, cracker, croissant or cream cake is then mopped up by insulin and sent packing into the brain and muscle cells for energy, with the excess sent to the fat cells to be stored as fat.

CHRONIC CARBI-VORE

Our love of carbohydrates – breads, pasta, rice, oats, crackers, cakes, biscuits, chocolate bars – comes from the heady rush of sugar that swiftly follows the ingestion of these highly palatable foods. The glucose high is enthusiastically mopped up from the bloodstream and presented to the cells of the body to use for fuel. This sees us going from the dizzying heights of our sugar bliss to the plummeting lows of DON'T. TALK. TO. ME. UNTIL. I'VE EATEN.

Our delight for sweet food comes from our drive to survive. Yes, you can thank your determined caveman genes for rearing their muffin-loving heads every time you try to resist the smell of freshly baked croissant, teasing your olfactory nerve as it shortcuts its way to the Fred Flintstone lurking inside your two-million-year-old brain. This sweet tooth would have served its purpose in the days of our land-dwelling ancestors. Access to the occasional bush of seasonal, sweet, juicy berries would have been a draw for our sugar-loving palates.

However, the endless shelves of packaged, artificially sweetened, highly processed and highly addictive foods that grace our modern-day food environment require us to become deafened to the incessant demands of our caveman genes as they go into a near frenzy, screaming at the top of their voices that we must stockpile more of this sweet stuff. As we give in to these deep-set DNA desires, we feel our health spiralling downwards and our desire for the sweet stuff sky-rocketing.

Our primal blueprint does not require us to feel hungry, to deprive ourselves of the pleasure of eating. A drive to eat is buried in our genetic wiring. It's in our survival manual, just like our drive for sex, to reproduce and pass on the parcel of our genetic code. We are wired to be rewarded when we eat. Dopamine is the heady hormone produced when we eat that bathes our brain in feel-good vibes, encouraging us to eat again, ensuring we don't starve to death. It's a potent self-reward system that can work *for* us or *against* us in the wrong food environment, in the same way that our genetic sweet tooth can. However, this self-reward system can become dysfunctional.

Have you ever noticed how one biscuit used to 'hit the spot' but it now takes half a packet for the same effect?! (Seriously, how does that happen!?! Jaffa Cake wizardry …) That desensitisation of our reward system demands you eat more and more Jaffa-liciousness to evoke the same heady high, and this can result in an overwhelming, uncontrollable urge to eat, to devour … a total eclipse as we seek out the dopamine rush. That dopamine high, coupled with the accidentally acquired status of a professional sugar-burner, almost guarantees that a sugar addiction ensues. So, if you find yourself a slave to the sweet stuff, in a narcotic Nirvana induced by nachos, bagels and biscuits, start by giving yourself a break. Your brain chemistry and caveman genes have been working against you! Your body does what it needs to do to survive and, in this case, it thinks that the aisles and aisles of cakes, biscuits and pastries are the equivalent of a life-saving buoyancy aid.

So, you need to release yourself from this sticky mess and stop your sugar-ravaged brain's destructive rampage. This isn't easy – sugar is addictive! But it *is* possible and it starts with balancing out brain biochemistry. Empowering alternatives to sugar create an easier transition to change. Levelling our metabolic hormones to switch on fat-burning and normalise appetite, and balancing gut bacteria and blood sugars allows for this to be a permanent lifestyle change, not just a diet. It becomes a way of life. You will dig yourself out of the rubble of the rubbish that gets marketed at us, which serves us nothing but chronic illness on a plate full of false hope and misery. You will emerge loving the feelings of unbridled control, working with your immense biological forces and feeling victorious.

So, what if you are already minding your sugars, conscious of your carb load and still struggling with weight, hunger and hormonal imbalance? There is more to this mystery than the sweet stuff alone.

How Stress Stores Fat

You have two little glands sat on top of your kidneys called the adrenal glands and their primary job is to try to keep you balanced. They are the internal reactors to any changes in circumstance that could cause harm to the body and they react by producing a cascade of stress hormones to help protect us from potential threats to our survival. Regardless of how well you are eating, if you are living in a state of stress and flogging your poor adrenal glands, your health will suffer!

Of course, some stress can be beneficial; it is the chronic, unremitting stress that is damaging to our health and can result in insulin resistance, hormonal disruption (and all of the associated symptoms), weight gain, anxiety, depression, cravings, insomnia, fatigue and feeling flat.

YOUR IN-BUILT DE-STRESS SYSTEM

Our in-built de-stress system releases cortisol and adrenalin, which govern and manage the stress response, causing a series of helpful physiological changes that you may recognise from a time when you felt a little under pressure – such as during an exam, a driving test or perhaps public speaking. This is known as our fight or flight state. Our heart rate jumps up a notch, blood flow is shunted away from our digestive system, kidneys and liver, and is directed to the muscles in preparation to flee from danger. Natural painkillers are released and fat is freed up for energy, our senses become heightened and we are ready for action. This doesn't sound too bad, more like a She-Ra version of our everyday selves! However, this is our response to a *short-term stress*, the one that makes us more robust and resilient. It is the *persistent* presence of long-term stress that causes a very different reaction in our body.

Persistent stress produces increased levels of the stress hormones cortisol and adrenalin. So while these are helpful hormones in short bursts, one of cortisol's primary jobs is to increase blood sugars, so persistent stress leads to persistently high levels of blood sugars, which in turn sees our insulin levels creep up. This sucks if you're staying away from the sweet stuff and here is your body making blood sugars in response to what it perceives to be a life-threatening situation you must flee from!

Where does it get this store of sugar? Does it use the store of fat on your body? Oh no, it breaks down muscle, which the liver helpfully converts into sugar. Not ideal when muscle plays such a big role in keeping our metabolic rate up high. What replaces that lean mass of muscle? Body fat. So, chronic stress leads to muscle being broken down into blood sugars, which is converted into fat and stored on our belly and can also lead to insulin resistance, making it really hard to lose that extra weight. Before you get stressed about that, get motivated, because we are going to be focusing on a diet and lifestyle that lower cortisol and optimises our 'rest and digest state'.

Yesssssss … ahhhhh.

SAVE OUR SEX HORMONES

Our sex hormones are sending out an SOS on a monthly basis via the symptoms we ladies have become only too accustomed to. The chronically high levels of blood sugars that accompany chronic stress have major implications for our long-suffering sex hormones. Reproduction is literally at the bottom of the to-do list when our body believes we are about to be eaten by a sabre-toothed tiger. Resources destined for reproduction are instead prioritised elsewhere.

Chronic stress is exhausting, it affects our sleep quality and sends our sugar cravings through the roof. At a time when we are least able to deal with yet more sugar surging through our bloodstream, here comes the comfort chocolate and the get-me-through-the-day digestives. If blood sugars are high enough for long enough, insulin resistance can kick in, which is not good news for our fertility or hormone balance. PCOS is a classic condition driven by insulin resistance (see Chapter Two) and the symptoms of perimenopause and menopause are intensified and prolonged in the presence of insulin resistance.

OI, CORTISOL, LEAVE MY PROGESTERONE ALONE!

Cortisol not only raises your insulin levels, switching on 'fat storage' mode, but also robs you of your keep calm and carry on hormone, progesterone. In Chapter Two we looked at the importance of progesterone in balancing out oestrogen's dominant ways. Cortisol is essentially made out of the same precursor molecule as progesterone, so when the demands to make more cortisol increase, progesterone becomes the fall guy. Chronic stress depletes our progesterone levels. Major stress during our menstrual cycle can impact fertility as ovulation becomes disrupted and the resulting corpus luteum (essentially a temporary progesterone-producing gland that appears following ovulation every month) produces low, suboptimal levels of progesterone.

Our body perceives all stress as the same: a threat to survival. Overtraining (particularly in the follicular phase), fasting for too long, infection, inflammation and nutritional deficiencies are all stressors signalling to the body that fertility comes second and survival comes first!

HOW SUSTAINED STRESS WREAKS HAVOC ON YOUR ADRENAL GLANDS

The stressors that we are persistently exposed to in our modern life cause our adrenal glands to be switched on far more than they are designed to be! Our constant stressing and worry see our two-million-year-old brain kicking into 'flee the tiger' mode on an hourly, if not continuous, basis and cause the overworked adrenal glands to become fatigued.

It is essential that we address this chronic stressed state, as our overworked adrenal glands will take over from our retiring ovaries come the late stages of perimenopause. If we don't look to build a robust and resilient nervous system, taking care of our adrenals, the transition from perimenopause to menopause can be frustrating and challenging.

It is worth remembering that stress is cumulative, and that includes all forms of stress, but particularly emotional stress. Often perimenopause becomes the time when these cumulative stressors reveal themselves. Unresolved trauma in the form of physical or sexual abuse, family conflict or highly emotional events can all lead to increased levels of cortisol via a nervous system that has been trained from a young age to be on high alert. Often this trauma is normalised or suppressed through coping strategies, such as comfort eating, drinking, drug-taking or other destructive behaviours.

Symptoms of overworked adrenals include:

— Excessive thinking
— Insomnia
— Feeling tired after waking up
— Brain fog
— Low tolerance to stress
— Susceptibility to infection and recurrent illness
— Reduced libido
— Weight gain and altered body shape
— Anxiety
— Depression

Chronic stress can leave us feeling increasingly anxious in the absence of sleep-inducing, calming progesterone. We can often end up feeling physically tired, yet mentally wired and unable to sleep. Chronically high levels of the stress hormone cortisol lowers our sleep hormone melatonin. The absence of high-quality sleep becomes yet another domino to fall in the disruptors to our hormonal balance, health and wellbeing.

Sleepless Is the Battle

Sleep might seem like something we do to rest our weary bodies, and that is correct, however, sleep is SO much more than an opportunity to recharge our batteries.

Sleep is highly influenced by our circadian rhythm, the biological changes the body goes through in a 24-hour cycle. Energy peaks at appropriate times of the day; you feel awake and refreshed in the morning with energy to carry out movement, focused work and tasks, then by the evening you beginning to feel calm, sleepy and ready for rest. Hunger levels are appropriate, too, gut health functions well and our health flourishes.

Sadly, much of how we live influences our circadian rhythm in a negative way, impacting our sleep, energy and hormonal balance. Minor changes to when and what we eat, how we sleep, levels of light exposure in our day and evening can all be highly influential on our sleep, weight, energy levels and long-term health.

SLEEP AND HORMONES

A number of beneficial hormones are released while we sleep. Melatonin, a key sleep hormone, is produced in response to darkness and supressed when we expose our eyes to light. Melatonin eases us off to sleep, but also possesses anti-inflammatory and antioxidant properties. Melatonin is made from our feel-good hormone, serotonin. Low oestrogen lowers serotonin which in turn can impact sleep through lower levels of melatonin.

Growth hormone is another important hormone that is produced while we sleep. As a child, growth hormone does as it says on the tin: it helps us to grow. As an adult, growth hormone is used to preserve proteins, hair, skin, nails, cartilage, muscles – it is the ultimate anti-ageing hormone! It also helps to build muscle and stokes your metabolic fire and fat-burning machinery.

Women lose growth hormone at an earlier age than men, resulting in women being more prone to muscle loss and, sadly, weight gain. The loss of growth hormone makes us more prone to insulin resistance (there is more blood sugar and less muscle to use it up). From the age of forty-five to fifty this decline can see us gradually gain resistant weight as muscle is replaced by body fat.

WHAT DECREASED GROWTH HORMONE?

Chronic stress, insomnia and increased sugar consumption can all lower growth hormone levels. Optimising sleep can increase growth hormone levels, leading to improved lean muscle mass, insulin sensitivity and weight status.

A poor night's sleep will also disrupt insulin sensitivity, meaning that when you do eat food with a higher carbohydrate load, your body is less able to mop up the blood sugars and more likely to convert them to fat. The hunger hormone ghrelin increases following a poor night's sleep and levels of 'I'm full' hormone leptin become lower. This double whammy means we are more likely to overeat when we're not sleeping well.

Following a night of tossing and turning, cortisol levels rise, stealing yet more progesterone building blocks, disrupting our sex hormone balance and further adding to our inability to get good shut-eye.

There are many causes of poor sleep quality and insomnia. Many women experience insomnia as a result of low progesterone, which can happen at the beginning of perimenopause or during times of high stress. When our nervous system is stuck in a persistent state of fight or flight, overthinking, worry and obsessive thoughts can prevent sleep. Changes in work habits, particularly working from home, have blurred the lines between home and work life. Eating too late at night, alcohol consumption, too many stimulants such as caffeine and sugar during the day, physical inactivity and too much exposure to light before bed can all impact the quality and quantity of our sleep.

Optimising sleep can be *transformative* for hormonal health, energy, body composition and long-term health. The third principle covered in this book will be dietary and lifestyle habits to optimise sleep, a foundational pillar of hormonal balance.

Overfed and Undernourished

Most diets fail because they don't address what drives hunger, what drives us to eat. The command that sees our hand come to our mouth in such a way that it seems out of our control … How is it possible to be so determined one day and the next find yourself hoovering a whole packet of chocolate buttons like you're in a competitive eating contest? Many people feel like a failure, feel shameful when they try and try, time and time again, to lose weight, turn over a new leaf and then blame themselves when it fails, beating themselves up for their lack of willpower. Or, worse, they give in, accept the status quo and see themselves slip further into a downward spiral or depression, failing health and premature ageing.

How do we break the pattern? How do we normalise hunger hormones, reduce cravings, improve insulin sensitivity, increase fat burning, improve energy and motivation, balance sex hormones and create lasting health? How do we stop fighting our biochemistry and start working with our physiology?

A nutrient-dense diet is a must for hormonal balance. A diet that ensures we prioritise the nutrients and building blocks required to support the needs of our bodies as they go to battle with the challenges that we face on a daily basis. Fuelling our body with great nutritional armoury is the first step to helping create balance in our busy lives. Chronic stress burns through our nutrient reserves, depleting us of the key nutrients magnesium, zinc and vitamin C. Food is not simply fuel, it provides the building blocks for our entire body – from our bones, muscles, skin, hair and nails, to the enzymes and compounds needed to drive the biochemical reactions. Sex-hormone building, balanced brain chemistry, sleep hormones, metabolic compounds, they all require *key nutrients* to function. Without the correct building blocks we simply cannot make the biological messengers needed for our internal chemistry work as it should.

Healthy fats form the backbone of our hormones. Nutrients are needed for our feel-good brain biochemistry, amino acids are essential for building strong, thick hair, nails, skin, bones and cartilage. A foundation of food-based nutrients with a selection of key supplements to boost levels and support the body in times of stress and additional needs can see our health transform.

Chapter Four will focus on food as the foundation for optimal hormone balancing, happiness and health. Specific nutrients, supplements, herbs and botanicals support this journey to optimal health.

Move It

We all know that we should move a little more and sit a little less. However, there are some simple core principles that we can incorporate into our everyday life that can transform sleep, anxiety levels, mood, energy, hormones and weight. Simple daily habits that will see you spending more time in nature and not necessarily in a gym (unless that's your thing, but we still need to make time for some daylight in our life!).

Spending time in nature might sound like I'm about to break out into a chant and instruct you to start burning joss sticks, but please, bear with me. While time in nature might not be at the top of your list of things to do to balance hormones and regain your shapely curves, believe me, it would be remiss of me not to include this as a principle within this book. It is a *powerful* stress reliever, sleep builder and hormone balancer, and much of it comes down to our exposure to light and getting moving.

When we expose our eyes to daylight first thing in the morning, a clear signal is sent to every cell in the body, communicating that it is time to become alert, motivated and ready for whatever the day brings.

Wakefulness is coordinated by a series of neurotransmitters, that are released upon exposure to daylight, vitamin D and with the presence of key nutrients. Upon waking, a natural spike in cortisol, serotonin and dopamine levels increase to heighten alertness and motivation. Serotonin, whose activity is increased upon exposure to daylight and decreased with reduced exposure to daylight, is associated with arousal from sleep, alertness, satisfaction and mood. Serotonin is converted to melatonin later in the day which supports restful, quality sleep. Therefore, optimal levels of serotonin are also associated with good sleep and low levels with insomnia. Low levels of vitamin B6, vitamin D, folate and the amino acid tryptophan are associated with low levels of serotonin. While this offers an overly simplistic view of what is required for serotonin synthesis, without fulfilling the fundamental basics mentioned above, we are starting off at a disadvantage! *Exposure to daylight and key nutrients are needed for optimal levels of serotonin.*

Scheduling in a morning walk to your daily habits has an extraordinary number of benefits to overall health and wellbeing. The light exposure helps to set your internal body clock, communicating the time of day and how awake and alert, or tired and sleepy you should be feeling. Exposure to daylight also stimulates a hormone called melanocyte stimulating hormone, which suppresses and regulates our appetite (have you ever noticed you feel less hungry in sunny climates or when you spend lots of time outdoors?) and increases our sex drive.

Walking outdoors not only exposes our body to daylight, setting our vital internal clock, it also has an interesting impact on a part of the brain that regulates fear, the amygdala. A simple walk can lower stress levels, alleviate anxiety and build on our 'courage' pathways according to neuroscientist Andrew Huberman. When we walk, jog or cycle or engage in any form of self-generated forward propulsion, our eyes scan the landscape in a side-to-side motion, ensuring the pathway ahead is clear. This forward motion with 'eye scanning' has a calming effect on the amygdala, the fear centre of the brain. The eyes are effectively communicating to the brain that the 'coast is clear of danger', generating a feeling of calm and relaxation.

There is a bonus prize for this morning stroll and taking in the scenery – the 'eye scanning' and forward motion also fortify the feeling of 'courage and boldness' through activating winning circuitry in the brain. Win-win.

When we start the day with a walk, it sets the scene for the brain, evoking wakefulness, alertness, calm, courageousness and feelings of boldness. Couple this with the benefits we all know so well, the importance of movement for muscle building, balance, strong bones, improving blood sugars and cardiovascular health, and that simple stroll in the morning is starting to look like a life-saving activity!

Combine that daily walk with a low-insulin lifestyle, reduced stress, better sleep, nutrient-dense diet and soon those small steps every morning become a giant leap forward in the direction of better physical and mental wellbeing and self-kind.

Four

Habits for
Hormonal Balance

OK, so we've run over some basic biology 101, we know the importance of keeping our sex hormones in check and why they become imbalanced, so now it is time to connect the dots. Having identified the disruptive patterns of modern eating and lifestyle, the principles of working with your female physiology are dovetailed with recipes and practical protocols that are here to guide you to hormone harmony.

Living La Vida Low-carb

A low-carb approach really goes hand in hand with a low-insulin lifestyle. As previously mentioned, it is not diet alone that drives our insulin levels up, so living a low-insulin lifestyle is a better principle to follow than focusing on the impact of food alone.

BE A CONSCIOUS CARB-EATER

Carbs are not the enemy; it is our over-reliance and chronic consumption of carbs and our long-drawn-out window of eating that cause our blood sugars to rollercoaster through the day. Becoming conscious of the foods that most impact our blood sugar and those that help to keep blood sugar spikes down, insulin levels low and optimise fat burning is important.

A continuous blood glucose monitor can help you to see on an individual basis which foods will impact your blood sugar the most, however, as a general approach, these include:

— Foods highly sweetened with sugar
— Processed foods high in sugar and fat
— Wheat products
— Grains

61

While wheat products have a surprising impact on our blood sugar levels, this does not mean no bread, cakes and biscuits; it means finding alternative options that do not send our blood sugar levels rocketing. In time, your palate may adapt to lower levels of sugar, meaning less sweetener is needed, however, there are sweeteners that have less of an impact on our blood sugars, which will be discussed in Chapter Five.

HOW MANY CARBS SHOULD I BE EATING PER DAY?

This is not an easy question to answer because we all have different levels of glucose tolerance – that is, some of us look at cake and gain weight, while others never seem to gain weight. Insulin resistance has a big impact on our ability to mop up blood sugars. If you've had many years of emotional stress, eating a high-carbohydrate diet, sleeping poorly, are over the age of forty and have a fairly sedentary lifestyle with some resistant weight to lose, your carb intake may need to be lower than someone who is highly active with high glucose tolerance.

As a guide, look to get most of your carbs from starchy veg (more on this in the next chapter) and aim to eat under around 50g carbs per day. However, counting is not necessary if you are sticking to the principles of grain-free (which cuts out wheat products), plenty of veggies, quality protein and moderate heathy fats. Remember, insulin slams on the brakes of fat-burning, so understanding the impact that foods have on your blood sugars is key!

Time-restricted Eating

Time-restricted eating is a very effective way of increasing insulin sensitivity, stimulating fat burning and losing weight, regulating hunger hormones, improving blood sugar stability, encouraging better-quality sleep and reducing cravings. The research of Dr Satchin Panda, author of *The Circadian Code*, suggests that when you eat is even more important than what you eat, for weight loss and wellbeing.

Time-restricted eating allows blood glucose levels and insulin levels to lower to a point where fat-burning is stimulated. Finding a window of eating that works for you and consistently sticking to it can be a game changer! Ideally, our window of eating would start in the morning and finish by early evening. Eating too close to bedtime can impact melatonin levels (our sleep hormone) which begin to rise around two to four hours prior to bed.

A typical time-restricted window may look like:

— **Breakfast**: 8am

— **Lunch**: 1pm

— **Evening meal**: 6pm

This ten-hour eating window should include all meals, snacking and calories. Only water and herbal teas would be consumed outside of this window. If you are having an alcoholic drink such as a glass of wine, either having it before your meal or during will keep it within your eating window. Time-restricted eating also increases the levels of growth hormone – key for muscle building and keeping metabolic rates high.

Time-restricted eating should be discussed with your doctor if you have any underlying medical condition, such as diabetes, or you are underweight.

Snack Attack

Desserts and healthy sweet treats should ideally be consumed after your meal. Fibre from vegetables helps to lower the impact of higher-carb foods on our blood sugars. If you fancy a snack during the day, keep it in your window of eating, not afterwards. The occasional snack when out with friends or at a celebratory event works, however, consistency is key! Ditching the evening snacks is transformative – try it, it works!

It may take a little time to adjust to this new regime – especially if you've been used to evening snacking. We have a lot of subconscious associations with relaxing in front of the TV with snacks or chilling out with a glass of wine in the evening. Try to replace old habits with new empowering ones, such as a walk after dinner, drinking various herbal teas for relaxation as well as the health benefits, or listening to music or reading. Sometimes a habit as simple as cleaning your teeth after you've finished eating your evening meal can help create the signal that the kitchen is now closed and you're done eating! It can take a little time for the hunger pangs to normalise; our body becomes trained to produce hunger hormone spikes when we consistently eat at a certain time, so if 8pm is your usual snacking time, that's when you'll get a bump in ghrelin hormone telling you to eat! This passes within a few days, so keep to it!

Prioritise Protein

We want to retain and build muscle. Look, I'm not suggesting you head out to your local gym to pump iron (although that could be a game changer!), what I'm saying is muscle is your BEST friend, your cheerleader when it comes to ramping up your metabolism, mopping up blood sugars and maximising metabolic health (as well as improving strength and balance). Muscle is the main insulin-sensitive tissue in the body. The more muscle we have, the better our insulin sensitivity and more able we are to burn fat and keep rising blood sugars at bay!

Protein must be consumed in high-enough amounts to retain and build muscle. There is a growing reluctance to eat protein from animal sources, and if you choose to not do so for ethical reasons, examine alternative sources. However, animal sources of protein offer the highest level of protein, incorporating a range of other important and valuable nutrients, too. While there are meat-free options within the recipe section of this book, red meat, fish, eggs and healthy sources of dairy are frequently seen within the recipes as superb sources of protein and other prized nutrients. Sources of healthy protein are outlined in 'Fridge Staples' in Chapter Five.

Our need for protein increases as we age. Our ability to break down protein into its constituent parts – amino acids – reduces with age, so we need to ensure we are eating sufficient quantities of this nutrient, even supplementing protein powder or collagen peptides where necessary, to build muscle and maintain the structural integrity of our bones, skin, female reproductive organs (vagina wall), cartilage, hair and nails.

Protein is better digested when eaten with healthy fats, and protein and fat often come packaged together as seen in nature – within eggs, fatty fish, meat and cheese. Fat often gets a bad rap, but healthy fats are an essential nutrient that offers many benefits.

Have Healthy Fats

A moderate amount of healthy fats is important for optimal health. How much is moderate? This depends on how much fat you have to burn as well as your liver function and ability to process fat, and how physically active you are. When following a low-carb lifestyle, a balanced plate could typically have 50 per cent colourful, leafy, cruciferous veggies, 30–40 per cent protein and 10–20 per cent healthy wholefood fats and oils.

A group of fats, essential fatty acids, offer key health-promoting benefits to us as humans. As we age, there is an increased tendency for inflammation. Adopting an anti-inflammatory approach to eating is of great importance in reducing chronic inflammation. A diet rich in omega-3 fatty acids can help balance out the pro-inflammatory effect of too much omega-6 in our diet. The typical Western diet is very high in omega-6 and very low in omega-3 fatty acids. Fatty fish, eggs, linseed and sesame seeds are rich sources of omega-3 – which we will cover in Chapter Five.

Soothing a Stressed Nervous System

As discussed in Chapter Three, reducing chronic stress is essential for optimising hormonal balance, improving sleep, restoring energy, losing weight and for better long-term health. Long-term stress is comparable to smoking in its detrimental impact on our health. The body does not regenerate and heal well from a state of fight or flight, so lowering the stress hormones cortisol and adrenalin is a must for ensuring health and longevity.

Our dominant thoughts inspire our reality. What we think on a daily basis is building the life we live. So, let's look at some tools that we can easily incorporate into our daily habits that can lower stress, take us into our 'rest and digest' and out of our 'fight or flight' mode.

WHAT'S GOOD FOR THE BRAIN IS GOOD FOR THE BODY

Giving our body the nutritional tools to build a resilient, adaptable and high-functioning brain helps to fulfil one aspect of eating for hormonal harmony and happiness. After all, you will feel what your brain wants you to feel. If you're lacking, your brain will communicate that in many ways, from low mood to cravings, insomnia to chronic anxiety.

Many common symptoms of modern living can be improved by supporting the brain nutritionally, however this does not complete the picture. While this is an oversimplification of an extraordinarily complex structure, seeking ways to maximise and support the health of our brain is essential as we travel through our female lives. With the perimenopause representing such a great time of change in our hormonal landscape, this has a huge influence on our nervous system, too, heightened more with insulin resistance and inflammation.

How we wire our nervous system is just as essential as the food we eat when it comes to looking after our brain and soothing our nervous system.

We need to provide the brain with:

— The nutrients it needs to thrive
— Positive wiring of our response to the world in which we live

The nutrients our brain needs to function are essential for communication between brain cells (neurones), and to build the neurotransmitters (brain hormones) dopamine, serotonin and GABA (see page 67), to name a few, and to give the various areas of the brain optimum fuel to do their job. These potent chemicals make us feel happy and ready to burst into song in the shower (thank you, serotonin), motivated and energised (pretty dope, dopamine), sociable, bonded and loved (over to you, oxytocin), calm and relaxed (great job, GABA).

A diet rich in nutrients needed to synthesise the range of biochemicals influencing our everyday emotions is the foundation of this book. What is good for the brain is good for the body; in Chapter Five, you will find a list of foods essential for brain health as well as supplements for supporting brain chemistry.

The Insulin-resistant Brain

Brain fog, low mood, anxiety, feeling tired all the time, constantly hungry, irritable … these are some of the common complaints of women entering the perimenopause period (any time from thirty-five years onwards). An insulin-resistant brain exacerbates and prolongs the symptoms of perimenopause and menopause. Why? Oestrogen assists insulin in ushering blood glucose into the various areas of the brain responsible for hunger and temperature regulation, fear and anxiety, memory and rational thinking, so when oestrogen declines, it becomes more challenging for our brain cells to access glucose to do their job. Now if the brain cells are already in a state of insulin resistance from years of stress, a high-sugar, high-carb diet, nutrient deficiency (particularly magnesium – more on this later), the brain now faces a whole world of hard work to get fuel into the brain cells. Lower oestrogen and insulin resistance are very destabilising for the brain!

The brain goes through a recalibration process in order to adjust to changing oestrogen levels – this is perfectly normal. However, that recalibration can feel more like the floor dropping away if our blood sugars are out of balance, we have insulin resistance, a malnourished, nutrient-deficient brain and poor lifestyle habits. When we layer this scenario with the loss of calming, relaxing progesterone, you can begin to see why metabolic flexibility, the ability to use both glucose and fat for fuel, is key in restoring business as usual in the perimenopausal brain.

It is never too late to improve insulin sensitivity. In the brain, muscles and fat cells. A low insulin lifestyle is of great importance for the short-term and long-term functioning and health of our brains.

Building Robust Brain Chemistry

GO GAGA FOR GABA

GABA is a chemical compound found in the brain that promotes sleep, reduces feelings of anxiety and exerts a calming influence. Think about how it feels when you've had too few many coffees – that's the feeling of having too much excitatory brain chemistry and not enough GABA. This neurotransmitter is the cornerstone of calm in the brain; when we drink alcohol, the GABA pathway is targeted, making us feel chilled and relaxed. Low GABA levels are found in those with panic disorders, insomnia, anxiety, depression, bipolar disorder and alcoholism, and while this doesn't mean that low GABA has caused these conditions, it could be contributing to the overall picture.

Low serotonin, poor dietary habits and prolonged stress can all contribute to low GABA levels. Caffeine can also inhibit GABA release, as it competes for the GABA receptors, reducing the effects of GABA. I'm not saying don't drink caffeine, but maybe consider switching to a decaf if you suffer from anxiety, insomnia, panic disorders or you struggle to relax.

Vitamin B6 is needed in order for GABA to function – sources of B6-rich foods and specific supplements are further explored in Chapter Five. L-theanine is the precursor of GABA and can be taken as a supplement to calm and lower anxiety (see Chapter Five).

Magnesium acts in the same way as GABA does in the brain, facilitating a calming effect. As GABA levels decline with age, magnesium supplementation may become increasingly important in maintaining the benefits of GABA.

Other ways found to significantly increase GABA are through yoga breathing techniques, taking longer exhalations than inhalations. (For more information on breathing techniques, see *Breathe* and *The Oxygen Advantage* in the Resources on page 247.)

DO AS I SAY DOPAMINE

Dopamine shapes behaviour. We learn what we like through associative learning when dopamine is released. Dopamine is highly motivating, rewarding and pleasurable. Low levels of this hormone are associated with low social and mental stimulation, high emotional stress (cortisol), inflammation, low vitamin D, low B6 and folate (B9), low tyrosine (an amino acid) and low oestrogen.

SUNSHINE SEROTONIN

Serotonin is your satisfaction neurotransmitter; it helps you feel alert, awake and happy. Low levels of daylight, activity or high levels of cortisol and inflammation, alcohol, caffeine and smoking, low tryptophan (an amino acid), vitamin D, B6 and folate and low oestrogen can all lead to low serotonin. Depression, lack of motivation and insomnia are signs of low serotonin; this doesn't mean that low serotonin has caused these conditions, but it could be contributing to the overall picture.

OH, OH, OH OXYTOCIN

Oxytocin promotes good mood and feelings of belonging, bonding and sociability. It reduces inflammation and promotes wound healing. Oxytocin is released when we orgasm – the more oxytocin released, the more intense the orgasm. Go, team oxytocin!

Low social interaction, low oestrogen and high testosterone lower oxytocin. Low vitamin C, magnesium, taurine (an amino acid) and vitamin D also lower oxytocin. Feelings of aggression, anxiousness and low sociability are associated with low oxytocin.

Wired to Unwind

The recipes and lifestyle habits in this book provide the nutrient building blocks necessary for optimal brain chemistry. But providing these biological building blocks is only part of the picture. Our brain responds to the stressors it deems to be a threat to our existence, sending us into a fight or flight frenzy. Wiring our brains to become resilient to the modern-day stressors that threaten our peace of mind and long-term health is a crucial element in soothing the nervous system.

Too many of us are not living our dream life because we are too focused on living out the fears in our head, driving our nervous system into a constant state of high alert and stress. Many of us have trained our nervous system into the fight or flight state, and so we find it hard to relax, to switch off. We must ease the fear-centre of the brain and shift it from a state of fight or flight into rest and digest.

There are some tools we can use to do this (with more resources at the end of the book).

ADAPTOGENS

Adaptogens are herbal and botanical remedies that can help increase our resilience to stress. They have long been used in Ayurvedic medicine but are increasingly gaining popularity due to their safety and the lack of side-effects that are associated with pharmaceutical approaches. Adaptogens can be found in teas, as powders and as supplements. (Specific adaptogens are covered in the 'WhatSupp' section in Chapter Five.)

GET OUTDOORS

Walking in nature naturally increases our dopamine and serotonin levels. Sunshine will also stimulate vitamin D levels, essential for making feel-good neurotransmitters.

BREATHING

Breathing patterns tap directly into our nervous system, calming or exciting it. Breathing can be used to increase alertness and stimulate adrenalin. It can also be used to calm, relax and bring down heart rate. James Nestor and Patrick McKeown are authorities on breathing and I would highly recommend looking at some of their work (see resources on page 247).

Without adequate, quality sleep, the brain will function suboptimally. Chronic sleep deprivation has even been highlighted as a risk factor for Alzheimer's disease in women. We must sleep for our mental, physical and hormonal health!

Sleeping Beauty

Having discovered the disruptive nature of poor sleep, let's look at the key principles that can improve and optimise sleep quality.

— **A good night's sleep starts in the morning** – our morning walk, exposing our eyes to daylight upon waking, is the ideal way to set our body clock, increasing dopamine and serotonin levels in preparation for peak alertness and focus for the day.

— **Coffee o'clock** – coffee can be the first thing many people reach for when the alarm clock is ringing. Waiting ninety minutes before hitting the caffeine can help the brain naturally shift to an 'awake' state. Keeping caffeine to the morning can also be hugely helpful if you struggle to sleep at night. Caffeine has a long half-life and can stay in your system longer than you think! Decaf may be a better option for those using coffee as a means to 'get going' in the morning, stimulating your already taxed adrenals.

— **Break-fast** – break your fast with a nutritious, blood-stabilising brekkie. Protein in the morning works well for our muscle-building biology. The breakfast ideas in the recipe section of this book prioritise protein, which will keep you feeling fuller for longer and provide the building blocks for making your feel-good neurotransmitters, dopamine and serotonin.

— **Light me up ... dim me down** – daylight in the morning, ideally at lunchtime and in the evening, signals to our circadian rhythms the time of day and whether we should feel awake and alert or sleepy and calm. Modern living is a threat to great sleep, as we spend too much time away from natural light in the day and expose ourselves to too much blue light from screens in the evening and at night. Light emitted from screens and phones blocks melatonin production, disrupting sleep.

— **Control light levels** – try to get outdoors first thing for a fifteen- or twenty-minute walk every day. If you can't get outside, sit by a large window to eat breakfast and lunch or place your desk near a window instead. Try to maximise your light exposure during the day, then as the evening approaches, start to reduce your light exposure. Using blue-light-blocking glasses while working at a computer can help protect melatonin levels in readiness for sleep. Then when you go to bed, try to create a really dark room, because darkness stimulates melatonin. A sleep mask can be really helpful if you live in an urban area with many streetlights seeping dim light into your bedroom.

— **Stop thinking … !** – excessive thinking before bed can be a sign that your adrenal glands have been working overtime and your stress response is struggling to switch off. Foods rich in sleep-boosting nutrients and supplements to ease you off to a night of good slumber are covered in Chapter Five, as well as the nutrient-dense recipes in Chapter Six.

— **Create a sleep-positive bedtime routine** – a sleep-positive routine is setting yourself up for a good night's sleep. This might include a cup of herbal tea, soaking in a warm bath with Epsom salts or reading a book. Staying away from negative or overly stimulating TV programmes which can increase cortisol and adrenaline. Meditation can also help relax the body and mind before bed, increasing oxygen levels through deep breathing and helping to switch off excessive thinking.

Nutrient Dense and Delicious

A nutrient-dense diet ensures we have a vast range of vitamins, minerals, antioxidants, fibre and protein in order to support the complex range of biological systems and demands of the body.

Poor digestive health, low microbiome diversity and overgrowth of unfriendly bacteria can be a source of low-level inflammation. High levels of blood sugars and inflammation rob the body of important nutrients needed for optimal insulin sensitivity as well as hormone-building and immune function.

Gut health and liver function are two key areas of focus for hormone balancing and optimal health. The gut houses the microbiome, a collection of beneficial bacteria, microbes and yeast that works in a win-win relationship with the body when in balance. If diversity lowers (which happens with age) or good bacteria become crowded out by the bad, this can impact many areas of our health, including our oestrogen levels! Specific bacteria housed within the gut help to modulate oestrogen levels – who knew?

Adding a daily probiotic (bacteria-containing foods) such as fermented veggies (sauerkraut) and fermented drinks (kombucha, kefir) can help increase gut bacteria diversity and optimise overall health.

LIVER-LOVING FOODS

Our liver does more than just detoxify, it is one hardworking organ. The liver plays a crucial role in hormonal balance, ridding the body of 'used-up' oestrogen to allow room for new oestrogen to be made. This process happens in two phases, with each one needing key nutritional support and a well-functioning liver. A sluggish liver, arising from a high-sugar diet (resulting in fatty liver), alcohol and high toxin exposure and poor nutrient intake can result in hormonal imbalances. Used oestrogen cannot be adequately detoxified, leading to higher levels of circulating oestrogen.

Liver-loving nutrients, cruciferous vegetables, gut-happy tonics, teas and meals will add nutrients to optimise gut health, liver function, digestive health, hormonal detoxification and balance.

ALCOHOL AND HORMONAL BALANCE

Alcohol can impact some women more than others. If your liver is not working optimally, alcohol is likely to have a greater impact on you. Drinking alcohol with food is better than drinking on an empty stomach, however, you may find reducing your alcohol intake has great benefits for your sleep, blood sugars, liver function and hormone balance.

Movement

This is far more than jumping on a treadmill for thirty minutes; movement is an essential nutrient, a daily must. Movement does not have to mean going for a run or joining your local bootcamp group – one of the best forms of exercising is walking. Daily walking is at the top of the charts when it comes to life-changing habits – you can change the course of your health in such a big way. Layer that on top of time-restricted eating and a low-insulin lifestyle, and that's when you really start shifting gears.

Walking gets the big muscles working – the thighs and butt muscles – which use up a lot of glucose. Getting your legs moving ramps up your metabolic rate and helps build tone in those powerhouse muscles.

A walk after you've eaten reduces the blood glucose spike (such a simple habit!). Make a pact to incorporate walking into your day, starting with a morning stroll to stimulate your dopamine and serotonin, get daylight into your eyes (ideally walking without sunglasses, don't look directly into the sun) and set your circadian rhythm. The forward motion of walking (or jogging and running) also calms the fear-centre of the brain, lowering anxiety while leaving us feeling set up for the day.

A twenty-minute session of resistance exercise produces a boost in growth hormone, supporting muscle building and metabolic rate. Incorporating two or three sessions of resistance exercise into your week is a superb way of preserving and building lean muscle mass, improving insulin sensitivity and optimising overall health.

Aim for a low-insulin lifestyle

— Become conscious of your carbs
— Prioritise protein
— Have healthy fats
— Try time-restricted eating

Soothe a stressed nervous system

— Consider adaptogenic herbs
— Get outdoors
— Breathe to relax
— Prioritise sleep – a key nutrient for the nervous system

Optimise sleep

— Get walking – a good night's sleep starts in the morning
— Go easy on the caffeine
— Light in the day, dark at night
— Reduce over-thinking, try quietening the mind
— Create a positive sleep routine

Increase nutrient density

— Optimise gut health – fibre-rich, probiotic-rich fermented foods
— Eat anti-inflammatory foods – omega-3-rich foods, turmeric, ginger, garlic, brightly coloured vegetables, vitamin-C-rich foods, vitamin-D-rich foods, preferably grain-free and gluten-free
— Ramp up metabolic health
— Optimise liver and bile health – cauliflower, broccoli, cabbage, beetroot, avocado, pecans, mushrooms
— Lower alcohol intake to support liver health, sleep and blood sugars

Move it!

— Have a morning walk
— Get the legs working
— Walk after eating
— Practise resistance exercise for a growth hormone boost

Five

From Fridge to Fork

It's time to Marie Kondo the fridge and kitchen cupboards. Planning is a key component in overcoming sugar cravings and food addiction and creating lasting change. When temptation comes knocking, having a selection of healthy options to hand prevents old habits creeping back in.

FRIDGE STAPLES

Fermented food

A daily forkful of fermented food is the ideal way to add good gut bacteria to your microbiome. Packed with easy-to-digest fibre that feeds the good bacteria and helps these happy microbes set up camp in your gut, there are SO many delicious fermented foods to choose from.

Sauerkraut
This partially digested cabbage concoction is jam-packed with bacteria, prebiotics and lactic acid. I know it sounds as sexy as woolly socks, but this ferment really is the Agent Provocateur of fantasy food. It brings so much goodness to your gut and is a rich source of vitamin C, an important vitamin for building progesterone and making collagen. Make sure your sauerkraut is labelled unpasturised or raw.

Kimchi
Kimchi originates from Korea and is served as a traditional side dish of salted, fermented vegetables. It is deliciously spicy and packed with gut-beneficial bacteria.

Beet kvass

Beet kvass is a fermented beetroot drink packed with naturally occurring nitrates. These important compounds form the building blocks of nitric oxide (NO). Nitric oxide has many benefits for women's health, including improving sexual function and maintaining vaginal health. As we age, we lose greater ability to make NO. The flow of blood to the vagina is controlled by nitric oxide, so increasing NO levels optimises this blood flow, which is important for the health of vaginal tissue (and can improve orgasms). NO can improve sleep quality, reduce inflammation, improve bone strength, reduce bone loss and help protect against heart disease – so many reasons to bring beet kvass into your daily habits! The recipe for Beet kvass is on page 110.

Kefir

Kefir is a fermented drink that is traditionally made from cow's, sheep's or goat's milk. Dairy-free kefir options, including coconut kefir, are widely available. Choose a low-sugar, plain kefir that can be added to smoothies, salad dressings or desserts. (See Chapter Six for more ideas.)

Kombucha

Kombucha is a traditional fermented tea drink often found with a range of fermented botanicals, herbs and spices added for extra goodness. Beware of sugar content, which ideally would be 3.5g carbs per 100ml or less. Add 50ml of kombucha to sparkling water for a delicious tonic with significantly lower sugar.

Fermented soya

Miso, tofu, tempeh and natto are all traditional variations of fermented soya bean. Soya beans, like many other foods, contain anti-nutrients that can lower your body's ability to absorb nutrients. Fermentation removes some of the anti-nutrient compounds (phytic acid), enhancing the nutritional value and transforming it into a highly bioavailable, nutrient-rich food. Fermented soy is also a rich source of vitamin K2, an essential vitamin for strong bones, teeth and cardiovascular health. Soya beans contain phytoestrogens, hormone-like compounds found in many food products such as nuts, seeds, coffee, dairy, cabbage and apples. Phytoestrogens can help to regulate oestrogen metabolism (detoxifying oestrogen that our body needs to get rid of). However, too much soya could affect fertility and disrupt menstrual cycles.

Fermented soya-based foods, from organic, responsibly sourced and grown crops, can have a beneficial impact on gut health and as a source of amino acids, calcium, copper, selenium and vitamin K2.

Dairy

Dairy is a super source of protein and calcium. However, at perimenopause, when our immune system can become reactive, increasing levels of histamine, the protein in cow's dairy, could worsen the symptoms of perimenopause. Switching cow's products (which have A1 casein) to goat's and sheep's products (which have A2 casein, an easier protein to digest) can ease some of the digestive issues experienced at perimenopause. Butter, ricotta and cream have relatively little casein present.

Yoghurt

Yoghurt is a great source of beneficial bacteria, healthy fats, calcium and protein. Casein, the milk protein in cow's yoghurt, can be challenging for some to digest. Goat's and sheep's yoghurt may be easier to digest due to the different casein present. Choose organic dairy where you can, with the least number of ingredients. Dairy-free options such as coconut yoghurt are widely available.

Cheese

Cheese is a great source of protein, calcium, zinc and vitamins A, B12, K2. Nutritional values vary depending on the cheese. K2, an important vitamin for bone and cardiovascular health, is made from bacterial growth and fermentation. Mature cheeses such as Munster, Camembert, Stilton, Gouda and Roquefort have significantly higher levels of K2 than younger cheeses. Goat's and sheep's cheeses have a different fatty acid profile to cow's cheese, offering higher levels of medium chain triglycerides, a type of fat that is broken down into ketones by the liver and provides an alternative source of fuel to glucose. Aged cheese is a super source of tyrosine, an amino acid needed to make dopamine. The crunchy crystals found in aged cheese are clusters of tyrosine.

Butter

Moderate amounts of butter provide a rich source of nutrients, including a particular fatty acid called butyrate. Butyrate offers many health benefits, from increasing insulin sensitivity to lowering inflammation. Beneficial gut microbes can make butyrate, which is an essential source of fuel for the cells of the colon. Having a healthy gut microbiome to produce the necessary levels of butyrate for bowel health is essential. Almonds, apples, garlic and kiwi can all increase butyrate levels, supporting and protecting colon cells and bowel health.

Ghee

Ghee is an ideal fat for those with a mild sensitivity to dairy, as the majority of milk proteins have been removed. Trace amounts may remain, though, so avoid this ingredient if you have a serious dairy allergy. Ghee has a high smoke point, making it ideal for high-temperature cooking such as roasting.

Eggs

Eggs are the ultimate fast-food, packed with a full spectrum of nutrients, healthy fats and protein. A bowl of boiled eggs deserves a coveted spot in the fridge!

Mayonnaise

Mayonnaise brings many a dull dish to life. Opt for an olive oil or an avocado oil mayonnaise, which are packed with health-boosting benefits and anti-inflammatory fats.

Meat and fish

Unprocessed red meat is one of the most nutrient-dense foods on the planet. High-quality protein is an essential component of optimum health and consuming red meat, some chicken, fish and eggs ensures that not only do you get access to high-quality protein but a vast range of nutrients and omega-3 fatty acids (particularly in oily fish), too. Organ meat is an affordable and often underused part of an animal, with liver being an exceptional source of the active form of vitamin A, or retinol, which is essential for eye, skin and immune health, to name a few.

Bone broth

Bone broth is packed with the amino acids glutamine, proline and glycine that are required for building collagen, detoxification in the liver and making neurotransmitters. As a rich source of calcium, magnesium and potassium, bone broth is Mother Nature's multivitamin!

IN SUMMARY ... YOUR FRIDGE WANTS TO BE PACKED WITH

— Sauerkraut
— Kimchi
— Beet kvass
— Kefir
— Kombucha

— Yoghurt
— Eggs
— Mayonnaise
— Aged cheese
— Meat/fish

STORE CUPBOARD ESSENTIALS

Finding an empowering alternative to well-loved foods such as bread, pasta, cakes and cereal is a key component in making lasting change. There are so many wonderful low-carb alternatives to choose from; below is a selection of low-carb swaps.

REPLACE	HEALTHY SWAPS
Rice	— Cauli rice — Broccoli rice
Wheat Pasta	— Spiralised veggies — Bean pasta — Lentil pasta — Chickpea pasta
Cereal/Oats/Granola	— Grain-free granolas (homemade, see page 133 or Keto Hana, Raw Gorilla) — No-oat meal
Wheat Bread	— Grain-free breads — Grain-free rolls — Grain-free bagels — Grain-free pizza bases
Wheat or Rye Crackers	— Almond crackers — Linseed crackers
Sweets and Chocolates	— Dark chocolate (ideally above 90% cocoa solids!) — Seeds and nuts — Healthy snacks (see recipe section)
Crisps	— Kale crisps — Cheese discs (see page 239) — Cheese cubes (I use Monarch's Pure or Cheesies)

Rather than having a cupboard full of spices and condiments that never see the light of day, here is a small selection of dried herbs, spices, sauces and condiments that will be used many times throughout the recipe section of this book, allowing you to make delicious meals in minutes.

SEASONINGS

— Garlic-infused sea salt (I like Dorset Sea Salt Co.)
— Beetroot-infused sea salt
— Himalayan rock salt
— Coconut aminos (I use Cocofina)
— Noya – soya and gluten-free, fermented seaweed sauce

HERBS AND SPICES

— Dried mixed Italian herbs
— Curry powder
— Smoked paprika
— Ground cinnamon
— Ground cumin
— Ground ginger
— Mixed spice

FATS, OILS AND VINEGARS

— Balsamic vinegar (I use Willy's Organic Live Apple Balsamic Vinegar and Biona balsamic vinegar)
— Apple cider vinegar – raw and unpasteurised
— Avocado oil
— Extra virgin olive oil
— Coconut oil
— Butter
— Ghee

MCT OIL

MCT, medium chain triglycerides, are small fat molecules that are easily broken down into a form of fuel called ketones. Ketones are an alternative source of fuel to glucose for the brain and muscles, making MCT oil a great choice for those with varying degrees of insulin resistance. MCT is a natural laxative made from coconut oil and can be very helpful if you suffer from constipation. Start with a small amount, such as ½ teaspoon, to build up tolerance and avoid overly loose stools.

CONDIMENTS – GLUTEN-FREE

— Olive oil mayonnaise (for
   pure olive oil mayonnaise,
   I use Hunter & Gather)
— Avocado oil mayonnaise

— Mustard
— Raw basil pesto (made with
   100% olive oil, I use Seggiano)

JARS AND TINS

— Passata
— No-added-sugar pasta sauce
   (Seggiano do a great range)
— Coconut milk and cream (I love
   the richness of organic Cocofina

   coconut products)
— Curry pastes – so handy when
   you need a quick and easy meal!
   (R&G offer a superb range of
   no-added-sugar pastes)

NUT AND SEED BUTTERS

— Almond nut butter
— Macadamia nut butter
— Walnut nut butter

— Pumpkin seed nut butter
— Tahini paste – light and black

BAKING

— My favourite flours for baking
   with are coconut and almond,
   as they are high in protein and
   fibre and low in carbs. Ground
   linseed also makes a nutritious
   and fibre-rich flour
— Almond flour
— Coconut flour

— Golden linseed
— Psyllium husk – helps to
   bind ingredients together
   plus a super source of fibre!
— Erythritol – sugar alternative
— Baking powder (Doves Farm
   do a great gluten-free one)

OTHER

— Nutritional yeast – a superfood
   source of B vitamins
— Riced cauliflower (I like
   FullGreen)
— Sea buckthorn juice – high
   in vitamin C and omega-7
— Collagen peptides
— Bone broth powder
— Mushroom powder – Lion's

Mane, ideal for hormonal
balancing, mood and memory
— Dark chocolate (ideally 90%)
— Cacao powder – a super source
   of magnesium, adding chocolate
   goodness to smoothies, bites
   and bowls
— Raw chocolate (dark, low-sugar
   Ombar and Before Chocolate)

The Low-carb Lowdown

LOW-CARB VEGETABLES

— Artichokes
— Asparagus
— Aubergines
— Avocados
— Beetroot
— Bok choy
— Broccoli
— Brussels sprouts
— Cabbage
— Carrots
— Cauliflower
— Celeriac

— Celery
— Courgettes
— Cucumber
— Fennel
— Garlic
— Green beans
— Kale
— Leeks
— Lettuce
— Mushrooms
— Olives
— Onion

— Peppers
— Pumpkin
— Radishes
— Rocket
— Spinach
— Squash
— Swede
— Swiss chard
— Tomatoes
— Watercress

LOW-CARB FRUITS

— Apples
— Apricots
— Bananas (the greener
  they are, the lower
  in sugar)
— Blackberries
— Blackcurrants

— Blueberries
— Coconut
— Figs
— Grapefruit
— Kiwis
— Lemon
— Lime

— Melon
— Orange
— Pomegranate
— Raspberries
— Strawberries

Nutrient Know-how

A full spectrum of nutrients is essential to human health. Each nutrient plays its part in a well-orchestrated system exquisitely designed to allow us to thrive and not merely survive. Many individuals are living with chronic subclinical deficiencies, leading to an array of symptoms from poor sleep, low energy, skin problems and digestive issues to low mood and hormonal imbalances.

Nutrients are a key factor for a well-functioning body. How much we need varies from individual to individual. In fact, it varies daily for that individual depending on stress levels, exercise levels, whether they are fighting an infection, what they are eating that week, if they are sleeping. The variables are huge! Understanding some of the key roles of some of our main nutrients can help you to monitor your own nutrient intake and increase it in times when you feel your body may need more support.

VITAMINS

There are two classifications of vitamins: fat-soluble and water-soluble. The fat-soluble vitamins are vitamin A, D, E and K2.

VITAMIN A

Vitamin A is important for healthy vision, a healthy immune system, bone strength and the flexibility and elasticity of your skin. It helps keep you looking youthful!

Deficiencies can lead to night blindness and poor vision, dry eyes and poor thyroid function and skin problems such as acne, poor wound healing, dry skin and little bumps on the skin (that resemble chicken skin).

Sources include: Animal sources of preformed vitamin A include liver, eggs, ghee, butter and cheese. Plant-based sources of carotenoids include orange vegetables (butternut squash, carrots, sweet potato) and tomatoes.

VITAMIN D

Vitamin D is made through exposure of the skin to the sunshine and is essential for healthy bones and teeth and an important participant in blood clotting. It also plays a major role in immune function – all in all, a pretty important vitamin!

Low-level deficiency can result in susceptibility to autoimmune conditions and increased risk of infections.

Sources include: beef liver, oily fish, dairy, nuts and mushrooms.

VITAMIN E

Vitamin E is a powerful antioxidant that's particularly involved in protecting the precious omega fats in the cellular membranes from free-radical damage. Vitamin E enhances the benefit of omega-3 by reducing the likelihood of them becoming oxidised in your bloodstream. Vitamin E has anti-ageing and cellular protective properties and is a natural blood thinner.

Take under medical supervision if you are taking anti-coagulating drugs.

Deficiencies can mean reduced immune system, hot flushes and dry skin.

Sources include: sunflower seeds, almonds, hazelnuts, spinach, broccoli, avocados.

K VITAMINS

Sources of K1 include: leafy greens such as spinach and kale as well as broccoli, sauerkraut and pumpkin seeds. Vitamin K1 is important for blood clotting, while K2 works in synergy with vitamin D and calcium and orchestrates where calcium is deposited in the body. This is a very important function of K2, without it calcium could be deposited in breast tissue, arteries and organs and not in the bones and teeth where it is needed. It is also an important vitamin for making the fatty sheath that surrounds nerve cells.

Deficiencies of vitamin K1 are bruising easily and excessive bleeding from wounds.

Deficiencies of vitamin K2 are osteoporosis, dental cavities and unwanted calcification deposits in tissue.

Sources of K2 include: aged cheese, butter, ghee, eggs yolks and natto.

Sources of K1 include: kale, spinach, broccoli and Brussels sprouts.

WATER-SOLUBLE VITAMINS

These vitamins are not stored well in the body (with the exception of B12, which can be stored in the liver) and so they need replenishing regularly. Nutritional yeast (fortified with B12) is a good source of full-spectrum B vitamins.

VITAMIN B1 (THIAMINE)

B1 has the power to protect your arteries from high sugar and high insulin. It's also very important for the production of energy.

Deficiencies can show up on the nails as horizontal ridges. B1 deficiency leads to a build-up of a lot of nervous energy, where you just can't relax! Swelling in the calves and numbness in hands and feet, increased heart rate, anxiety, restless legs due to retention of lactic acid (B1 helps release the lactic acid), sea sickness or car sickness and nightmares are all signs of potentially low vitamin B1. Severe deficiency can result in a condition called beriberi.

Overconsumption of sugars – grains, sucrose, fructose and alcohol – can cause a deficiency.

VITAMIN B2 (RIBOFLAVIN)

Important in the regeneration of glutathione (the super antioxidant) as well as pathways involved in energy production.

Deficiencies can lead to headaches, depression, blood-shot eyes and cracked skin on the heels. A B2 deficiency can also show up as inflammation in the corner of the mouth (angular cheilitis) and a red tongue.

VITAMIN B3 (NIACIN AND NICOTINIC ACID)

This vitamin is important for the production of energy. It is also beneficial for lowering triglycerides and cholesterol.

Mild deficiencies can be seen as cracked skin on your heels.

VITAMIN B5 (PANTOTHENIC ACID)

Important for healthy adrenal function.

VITAMIN B6 (PYRIDOXAL 5'-PHOSPHATE)

An important vitamin for dopamine, serotonin and progesterone production.

Deficiencies can show up as redness around the nose and/or cheeks (rosacea), depression, low mood and poor mental wellbeing. A diet high in refined carbohydrates can cause a B6 deficiency.

VITAMIN B7 (BIOTIN)

Biotin is made by helpful bacteria in your gut. A gut microbiome imbalance can lead to lower levels of B7. Biotin is necessary for strong hair and nails.

Deficiencies can show up as weak, brittle nails, hair loss and thinning hair.

VITAMIN B9 (FOLATE)

Important for DNA production, a healthy immune system and energy production. Folate is found naturally in green leafy vegetables and citrus fruit. Folic acid is the synthetic form of this vitamin.

VITAMIN B12 (COBALAMIN)

Required for energy production and in the production of neurotransmitters.

A deficiency in B12 can lead to a sore, red, shiny tongue, with fissures (cracks) down the centre. It can also lead to neurological symptoms such as tingling in the feet (pins and needles), disturbed vision and an unsteady gait.

VITAMIN C (ASCORBIC ACID)

Vitamin C is essential for making collagen, the scaffold of the body (it prevents our skin from sagging). Poor collagen production results in slow wound healing, premature wrinkling, poor skin appearance, hair thinning and weak and brittle nails. Vitamin C is also a key nutrient for progesterone building.

Mild deficiencies can lead to bleeding gums, poor wound healing, spider veins and easy bruising.

Sources include: sea buckthorn juice is a high source of vitamin C. It is also a very rich source of antioxidants, carotenoids, bioflavonoids and omega-7, which can alleviate dry eyes and internal dryness. Sauerkraut, peppers, lemon, lime and kiwi are also good sources of vitamin C.

MINERALS

There are five major minerals needed for optimal wellbeing, these include calcium, potassium, sodium, phosphorous and magnesium.

CALCIUM

This is the most abundant mineral in our body, needed for strong, healthy bones and teeth. It is relatively easy to get calcium in our diets, with good sources including dairy, oily fish, greens, nuts, sesame and chia seeds.

Deficiencies in calcium can lead to muscle spasms, cramping and twitching, osteoporosis and poor dental health.

POTASSIUM

Potassium is an electrolyte, it can conduct electricity in the body and is needed in large quantities (4500–6000mg every day!). Why do we need that much? The sodium potassium pump that sits on the surface of your cells allow substances to pass in and out of your cells. You have rather a lot of these pumps and they require a lot of energy to run!

Deficiences in potassium can lead to muscle fatigue (heavy legs or lack of endurance) arrhythmia, fluid retention, low stomach acidity, muscle cramps and sugar cravings.

Sources include: leafy greens (kale, spinach, cavolo nero), avocados.

SODIUM

Sodium is an essential mineral – we need it to survive. We need about a ½ teaspoon of salt per day, which will provide us with sodium chloride. If you crave salt, it might be because you need it!

PHOSPHORUS

Found mainly in the bones, phosphorus is the second-most abundant mineral in the body. It is difficult to become deficient in phosphorus because it's in so many foods!

MAGNESIUM

This magnificent mineral is needed for the functioning of over 300 enzymes in the body. It has many roles, including stabilising blood pressure, energy production, muscle contraction and relaxation and strengthening the bones.

Why are we so deficient in magnesium?
There are many factors that influence magnesium levels, including alcohol intake, ageing, chronic stress, Crohn's disease, excessive calcium intake, heavy periods, high insulin, poor dietary intake of magnesium-rich foods,

poor gut absorption, strenuous exercise, uncontrolled blood sugars, vitamin B6 deficiency, vitamin D excess or deficiency and medications that can deplete magnesium. These medications include diuretics, digoxin, proton pump inhibitors, antacids and antibiotics.

The recommended daily allowance for magnesium is between 300 and 420mg per day, however, context matters. This amount will vary depending on your current health status, inflammatory levels, stress, exercise levels, dietary intake and the amount of sugar you eat (which depletes magnesium).

Why you can't skip magnesium if you're taking vitamin D

The recent interest in increasing vitamin D levels following the Covid-19 pandemic has seen high supplementation of vitamin D. However, high intake of vitamin D can deplete magnesium levels, therefore magnesium supplementation should be considered alongside vitamin D supplementation to minimise magnesium deficiency.

Symptoms of magnesium deficiency

Mild symptoms include anxiety, cramps (in the feet and hands), confusion, constipation, fasciculations (brief and spontaneous contractions of muscle fibres causing twitching under the skin), headaches, irritability, muscle weakness, tinnitus.

Severe symptoms include depression, hypertension, migraines and osteoporosis.

Magnesium-rich foods per 100g

— Pumpkin seeds 534mg
— Cacao powder 498mg
— Sesame seeds 351mg
— Brazil nuts 376mg
— Dark chocolate 327mg
— Almonds 268mg
— Black beans 160mg
— Mackerel 97mg
— Dark leafy greens – spinach, kale 79mg
— Basil 64mg
— Small avocados 58mg
— Bananas 27mg

Which magnesium supplement is best?

There are many different magnesium supplements on the market which vary in bioavailability.

— Magnesium salts or magnesium oxide – generally poorly absorbed.
— Magnesium citrate – draws water into the small intestine, loosens stools, can cause gastrointestinal upset. Ideal for constipation.
— Chelated magnesium – magnesium bound to an amino acid such as magnesium bisglycinate or magnesium glycinate. This magnesium compound is highly bioavailable, with a reduced incidence of gastrointestinal upset. The glycine may aid in sleep and is an important amino acid needed for building collagen. Glycine is also a key amino acid needed for building glutathione, a potent antioxidant made in the liver.

Individuals with kidney disease should supplement magnesium with caution as it could result in hypermagnesemia. Always seek professional advice before undertaking any new supplement regime.

Magnesium and women's health …

As our sex hormones change, so too do our inflammatory levels. Perimenopause sees inflammatory levels increase and an increased risk of insulin resistance and abdominal weight gain. Keeping inflammatory levels in check is key for a smooth transition from perimenopause to menopause. Low magnesium exacerbates inflammation and inflammation lowers magnesium levels. Insulin resistance also lowers magnesium, while magnesium deficiency drives insulin resistance.

Magnesium for migraines
Magnesium could help with migraine prevention as it inhibits the release of pain-promoting neurotransmitters while reducing neuroinflammation.

Magnesium for sleep
Magnesium supports the production of GABA, a calming neurotransmitter that makes you feel relaxed and chilled (this is the neurotransmitter stimulated with alcohol). Magnesium also lowers the stress hormone cortisol.

Magnesium B6 and PMS
Vitamin B6 is required for the maintenance of normal cellular magnesium levels. The combination of low B6 (or poor conversion to the active form P5P) and low magnesium has also been suggested to contribute to PMS, due to their dual role in synthesising bioactive chemicals, found to be deficient in PMS.

Polycystic Ovary Syndrome
PCOS is highly linked to insulin resistance. Low levels of magnesium can lead to insulin resistance, with insulin resistance further lowering magnesium levels.

Endometriosis
Endometriosis has an inflammatory component, with magnesium having an anti-inflammatory effect. Magnesium also has a role in relaxing smooth muscle, easing painful cramping.

Perimenopause, menopause and magnesium
Hot flushes have been associated with insulin resistance, high blood pressure and higher glucose levels. Evidence suggests that low magnesium is likely to be a contributing factor to hot flushes and night sweats, with insulin resistance and inflammation driving subclinical deficiencies.

Mood, mental health and menopause

Low levels of magnesium in women are associated with higher levels of depressive symptoms and higher levels of magnesium in women without depressive symptoms, indicating a greater vulnerability to depression in women with low magnesium intake.

TRACE MINERALS

Iodine, chromium, selenium, copper, manganese, iron and zinc are all trace minerals needed for optimum functioning of the body. We tend to be depleted in these because our soils are so drained of trace minerals, and thus so too the food from which it's grown.

IODINE

This is a vitally important trace mineral that's needed in very small amounts. It is important for thyroid function and for the health of the reproductive organs. It is also important for detoxifying heavy metals.

Deficiency in iodine can see you gain weight due to reduced thyroid function. Iodine plays an important role in balancing out excess oestrogen, and an iodine deficiency can lead to fibrocystic breasts and breast tenderness.

Sources include: Best taken as a food source such as organic seaweed or kelp supplements.

CHROMIUM

Chromium assists insulin in transporting blood glucose into the cells, improving blood sugar stability.

Broccoli has the most chromium of all the veggies; it's also found in beef and dairy.

SELENIUM

Selenium is a helper enzyme (a coenzyme) that's involved in the production of about twenty-five proteins. It is involved with making glutathione, a powerful antioxidant that naturally becomes depleted with age, stress, sugar and junk food consumption, when we have an infection or are exposed to lots of toxins.

Naturally found in Brazil nuts, meat and shiitake mushrooms.

COPPER

Copper helps form collagen and connective tissue, the scaffolding of the body, and it can help prevent premature greying of the hair.

Deficiency can lead to peripheral neuropathy (pins and needles in the hands and feet), loss of vision, a decrease in white blood cells, muscle weakness and anaemia.

Too much zinc reduces copper, so be cautious of over-supplementing zinc!

Sources include: organ meat, leafy greens, mushrooms, cacao.

MANGANESE

Manganese is important for making bone and connective tissue, so crucial for healthy joints, cartilage and bone health.

Sources include: cloves, pecans, pumpkin seeds and cacao.

IRON

Iron is the most common trace mineral deficiency. Absorbing iron is key to ensuring we are getting adequate levels in our body. Vitamin A, copper, zinc and vitamin C are necessary for optimal iron absorption. Calcium blocks the absorption of iron, so don't take a calcium supplement at the same time as eating your iron-rich food.

Deficiencies can make you feel pretty lousy, with symptoms ranging from hair loss, palpitations, low endurance, problems with concentration, shortness of breath, paleness, fatigue and weakness.

Sources include: liver, red meat, pumpkins seeds and leafy greens.

ZINC

Taking the oral contraceptive pill and a diet low in zinc-rich foods are common contributors of zinc deficiency.

Deficiencies appear in symptoms such as low mood, hair loss, skin problems – acne, eczema and rosacea, white spots on your fingernails could indicate a deficiency. Zinc can help lower inflammation associated with period pain and endometriosis and reduce vaginal dryness. Candida, a common fungal overgrowth, requires zinc in order to thrive. We compete with the fungus, in a nutritional tug-of-war over who gets the zinc. When candida wins, the immune system weakens as our zinc levels lower and the fungal infection thrives.

Sources include: oysters, meat, liver, pumpkin seeds.

ALPHA LIPOIC ACID (ALA)

This clever little antioxidant is both water- and fat-soluble. It plays an important role in making the super-antioxidant glutathione, recycles other antioxidants and is very important in glucose metabolism. It has been shown to help with diabetic neuropathies (damage to nerves due to high blood sugars). Human trials have shown improved blood sugars with increasing ALA.

Sources include: meat, liver, spinach and broccoli.

CO-ENZYME Q10 (COQ10)

CoQ10 is needed for the production of energy by our cellular batteries, the mitochondria. Low levels of the active form of CoQ10 can lead to fatigue. As we age, conversion of CoQ10 to the active form needed for energy production lowers. Certain medication, such as statins, can also deplete levels of CoQ10.

Sources of CoQ10 include: meat, poultry, fish, eggs and beans.

Heart meat contains high levels of CoQ10. As an important part of the energy-generating system and a potent antioxidant, heart meat or heart-meat supplements can support healthy energy levels.

INTELLIGENT FATS

Omega-3 fats are important for making hormone-type substances called prostaglandins. These are involved in blood vessel relaxation, boosting our immune function, water balance and pain and inflammatory pathways. New research is helping our understanding of how these intelligent fats improve our mental wellbeing, protect our brain from inflammation and neurodegeneration and improve focus and intelligence.

SOURCES OF INTELLIGENT FATS (OMEGA-3 DHA AND EPA)

Omega-3 rich foods – salmon, mackerel, herring, sardines, anchovies, eggs, grass-fed butter, ghee and meat.

High-quality fish oils – a high-quality, premium supplement is a great way to ensure you are getting the levels of omega-3 your brain needs to function. Cheaply produced fish oils could be rancid and could do more harm than good. Fish oils should be packaged in a dark bottle, wild, ideally Alaskan and processed in a way that minimises the opportunity to become oxidised. Select a high-quality, trusted brand.

Ahiflower – a sustainable agricultural crop grown by British farmers. Ahiflower seeds are pressed to produce a superior omega-rich, healthy oil. Due to its unique fatty acid profile, Ahiflower combines the health-support benefits of taking evening primrose, flaxseed and fish oils from a single plant, and is ideal for vegans, vegetarians and those seeking an alternative to fish oils.

WhatSupp

While food source nutrients are ideal, sometimes we need a little extra help from specific supplementation.

Please consult a health professional before undertaking any new supplemental regime.

SLEEP AIDS

— An adaptogen such as Ashwagandha: Try fermented Ashwagandha by Living Nutrition 600mg per capsule
— Magnesium bisglycinate (with/without tart cherry) such as Magnesium Complex or Smooth Mag by Terranova
— L-theanine and lemon balm

MOOD SUPPORT

— EPA – 500–1000mg. Choose a high-quality omega-3 fish oil such as Wiley's Finest Peak EPA or a vegan omega-3 rich in EPA such as Wiley's Finest CatchFree
— Vitamin D – 600IU daily
— Zinc – 8mg. Choose zinc citrate, zinc picolinate or bisglycinate
— B complex. Methylated B vitamins are ideal. BioCare and Terranova both offer excellent sources of methylated B vitamins

ADAPTOGENS

— Rhodiola – a traditional remedy to fight depression, anxiety and fatigue. Try Fermented Rhodiola by Living Nutrition
— Ashwagandha – can lower cortisol levels, promote quality sleep and potentially increase sex drive

ENDOMETRIOSIS – LOWERING INFLAMMATION

— Omega-3 fatty acids – anti-inflammatory
— Zinc – citrate or zinc picolinate
— Organic kelp capsules – to balance oestrogen

LIVER SUPPORT

— Milk thistle (fermented milk thistle by Living Nutrition is excellent)
— NAC – the precursor of glutathione, a key, potent antioxidant made
in the liver. Glutathione is especially important for those looking to
optimise liver function and lower free-radical stress

GUT HEALTH

— Digestive enzymes with food
— Betaine HCL with food
— Probiotics – Living Nutrition offers a range of high-quality probiotics.
Regenesis is ideal for restoring the microbiome following a course
of antibiotics

SKIN, HAIR, NAILS, BONE – TISSUES OF THE BODY

— Collagen peptides – 10–20g daily in smoothies, coffee or added
to food
— Bone broth powder – an alternative to making your own
— B vitamins – try Vitamin-B Complex with Vitamin C by Terranova
— Organ meat capsules – made with dehydrated liver, kidney and heart,
packed with a full spectrum of balanced vitamins and minerals. APE
Nutrition offer fantastic-quality organ meat supplements

LOW PROGESTERONE, OESTROGEN DOMINANCE

— Vitamin C – 1,000mg
— Selenium – 40–200mcg
— B6 – 30–50mg
— Zinc – citrate or picolinate
— Kelp – seaweed is a rich source of iodine, which can downregulate
oestrogen receptors, lowering oestrogen dominance. Organic kelp
supplements can help to reduce the symptoms of oestrogen dominance,
breast tenderness and endometriosis

PCOS – LOW OESTROGEN, HIGH TESTOSTERONE

— Optimise insulin sensitivity through diet, lower stress and
  optimised sleep
— Magnesium bisglycinate – try Magnesium Complex by TerraNova
— Zinc – can help with restoring hair loss, but this takes time!
— Spearmint tea

PMS & PERIOD PAIN

— Magnesium with B6 – relaxes contractions associated with
  painful periods.
— Smooth Mag (Terranova) is an ideal combination of magnesium
  bisglycinate and active B6 in a handy powder form to add to smoothies
— Omega-3 fatty acids – reduces inflammation
— Zinc – lowers inflammation.

HOT FLUSHES

— Magnesium with B6 – try Magnesium Complex by TerraNova
— Optimise insulin sensitivity and balance blood sugars

VAGINAL DRYNESS

— Try Wiley's Finest Orange Burst Omega-7 rich oil
— Zinc

HAIR LOSS

— Zinc
— B-vitamin complex
— Collagen peptides
— Vitamin C

BLOOD SUGAR CONTROL

— Magnesium bisglycinate
— Chromium
— Myo-inositol

SLUGGISH METABOLISM

Dietary

— ½ tsp–1 tsp daily MCT oil
— L-carnitine
— Omega-3 fatty acids

Lifestyle

— Resistance exercise two or three times weekly.
— Walk daily, start with a morning walk, before you eat (if suitable for you) will help increase fat burning.
— Walk after lunch, which can help keep blood sugars stable, keeping insulin levels down and increase fat-burning.
— Cold water exposure (if suitable for you, always follow guidance on getting started). Cold water showers are a good place to started. Cold water causes the body to work harder to warm up, using more energy. Cold water exposure, particularly cold-water swimming which sees the body immersed in cold water, increases metabolic rate and increases fat burning. This is due to an increased conversion of white body fat to the metabolically active brown fat.
— Time-restricted eating window – eating within a time frame of eight to ten hours can help to balance metabolic hormones, balancing blood sugars and increasing fat burning.
— Becoming conscious of your carbs. Reducing carb intake to a level that is appropriate for you. For some that may be under 50g per day. Don't get too focused on counting, just become conscious of the carbs you're consuming and the impact they have on blood sugars and insulin. Remember, insulin resistance will resist your best efforts to lose weight!

CONSTIPATION

Bowel movements can give us a good insight into the health of our digestive system! A daily bowel movement, with good consistency, can reflect a healthy digestive system. We do not want to be straining to have a bowel movement as this increases the pressure within our abdomen which can increase the risk of prolapse. Bowel movements contain toxins and metabolised hormones destined for disposal. If bowel movements are sat for too long in the bowels, waste products can be reabsorbed, with one such waste product being metabolised oestrogen. Experimental studies have suggested that women with healthy bowel movements are associated with a decreased risk of breast cancer due to healthier levels of circulating oestrogen. To support a healthy digestive system and healthy bowels, aim for one bowel movement a day (or more) with a snake-like consistency.

For optimal bowel movements

— **Get hydrated.** Dehydration can lead to constipation. Water-rich veggies and appropriate amounts of fresh water (with a slice of lemon for extra goodness) can support healthy bowel movements.

— **Get moving.** Sitting compacts our bowels, increasing the likelihood of constipation. Get up and walk around … sitting at a desk for too long is not great for our bowel health.

— **Fermented milk thistle** – this supplement aids bile stimulation and bile is very important for the easy passage of bowel movements.

— **Eat plenty of fibre-rich foods!** Fibre forms an important part of a healthy diet. Fibre helps to feed your gut microbiome as well as supporting the healthy passage of bowel movements. Fibre-rich foods such as apples, figs, spinach, cauliflower, linseed and chia seeds can all support healthy bowel movements.

— **Natural laxatives** – nature's natural laxatives can also support healthy bowel movements. Vitamin C is a natural laxative, found in sea buckthorn juice, citrus fruits, berries, bell peppers, sauerkraut or in supplement form such as liposomal vitamin C. MCT oil is also a natural laxative, start with a small amount (such as ½ teaspoon) as a small amount is very effective!

— **Magnesium citrate** – this magnesium compound draws water into the small intestine, which aids in loosening bowels.

— **Try a daily smoothie** – like Get a Move Along (see page 122).

Six

Recipes + Remedies

In this next section you'll find a range of low-carb, nutrient-dense and delicious recipes to suit all palates. You will notice that there is no wheat, grain or gluten in these recipes! There is an abundance of cruciferous vegetables … used in ways you may have never used a cauliflower before! You'll find plenty of protein and a range of vitamin and mineral-rich veggies and healthy fats. Whether you're a meat eater, vegetarian or vegan, there is something in this section for everyone.

Explore these recipes with an open mind and an air of curiosity … once you begin to experience the improved energy, better sleep, reduced cravings and food satisfaction from eating this way, your hungry brain will be happy, your hormones will become balanced and you'll be ready to start living your best life.

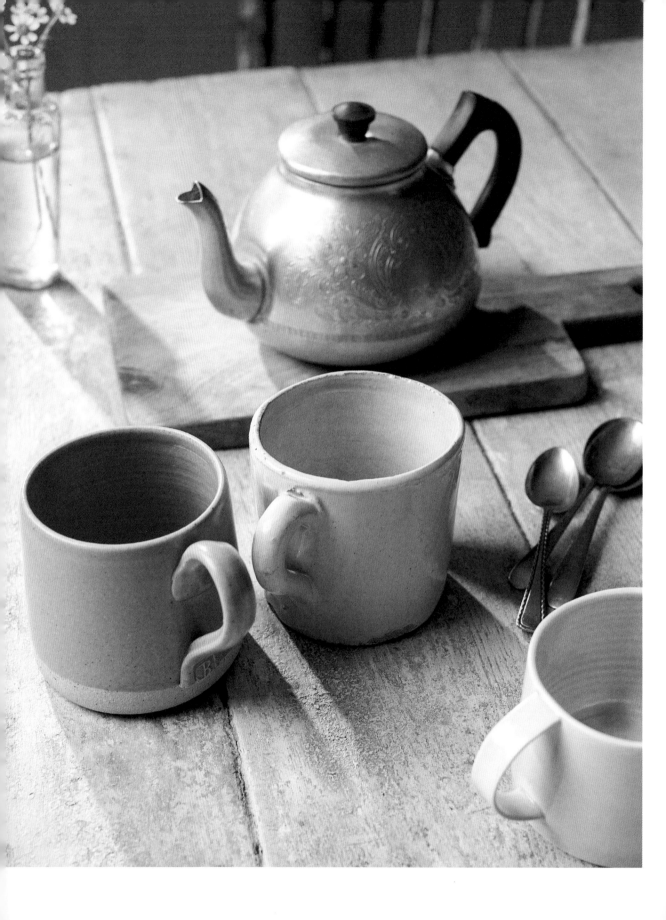

Teas, Tonics + Smoothies

Fat matcha

Matcha green tea is *very* high in antioxidants and has been linked to improvements in liver function, attention span and memory. Matcha can be consumed as a latte, or with a little twist …

1 mug of hot water
½–1 tsp matcha tea powder
1 tbsp collagen peptides
(optional)
½–1 tsp coconut oil, ghee
or MCT oil
1 tsp sweetener of choice,
such as erythritol or raw
honey (optional)

1. Add all the ingredients to a suitable heatproof blender (being mindful of the hot liquid when blending!) and whizz on a low setting until combined and frothy.

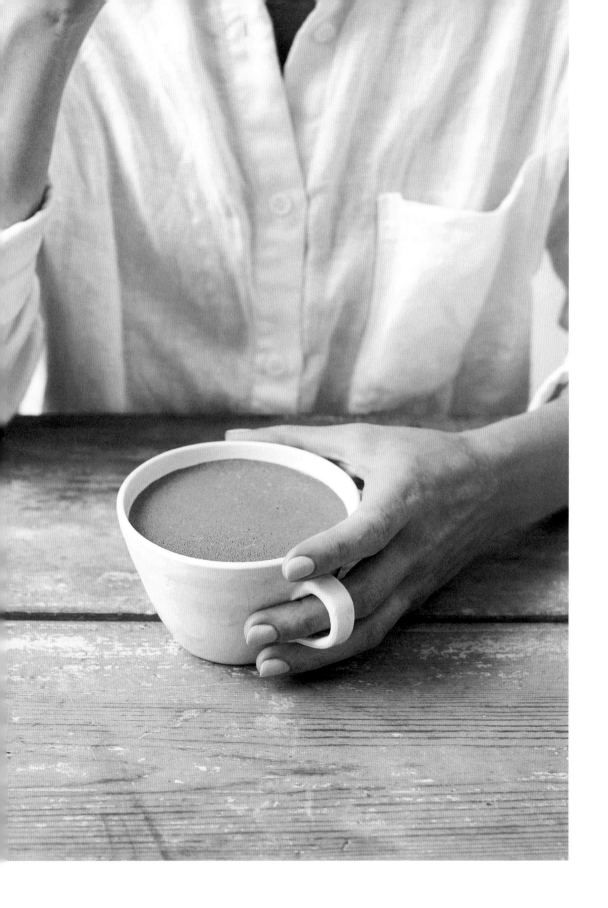

Horm-fix

This Horlicks look-a-like hot drink helps to
support oestrogen levels and ease you into
a good night's sleep. Smooth Mag is a blend of
melatonin-boosting Montmorency tart cherry,
calming magnesium and B6 (which supports
healthy progesterone levels), as well as blood-
sugar-balancing inositol.

1 mug of unsweetened hazelnut milk
1 tsp maca powder
½ tsp mushroom powder – I use Lion's Mane (optional)
2 tsp Smooth Mag (optional – see page 97)
½ tsp cinnamon

1. Add all the ingredients to a saucepan
    and warm gently, stirring occasionally,
    until well combined.

2. Transfer to a mug, stir to prevent the content
    settling at the bottom of the mug and drink.

(Photographed opposite)

Fat coffee

When you're looking for a breakfast to go that
won't impact your blood sugars, a fat-fuelled
coffee makes for a satisfying start to the day. With
the addition of mood-boosting mushroom powder
and skin-loving collagen, this coffee packs a punch!

1 hot brewed Americano
½–1 tsp MCT oil (see page 82)
1 tsp coconut oil or ghee (optional)
1 tbsp collagen peptides (optional)
½ tsp mushroom powder – I use Lion's Mane (optional)

1. Carefully empty the hot Americano into
    a heatproof blender, then add the rest of
    the ingredients and blend until frothy and
    well combined.

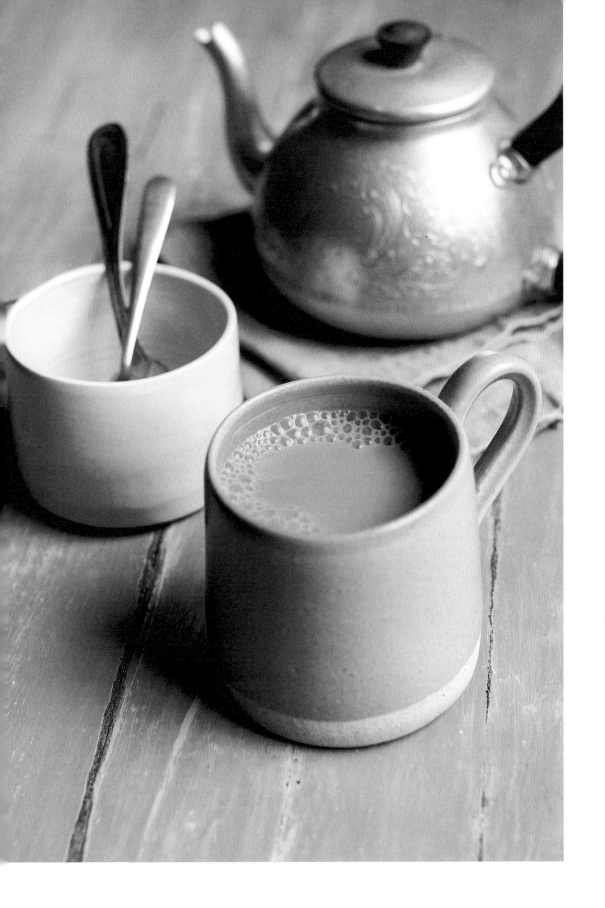

Beet kvass

This super juice ticks so many boxes – it's packed with beneficial bacteria, antioxidants and nitrates, and it's also a powerful tool for optimising many areas of health. Skin health, sexual function and cardiovascular health in particular, all benefit from the boost in nitric oxide that's obtained from a blissful beet kvass.

2 litres filtered water
20g fine Himalayan pink salt
4 medium unpeeled
    beetroots (ideally organic)

1. Clean the jars you are using with hot soapy water and rinse well.

2. Boil ½ litre of the water in a large saucepan and add the salt. Stir until fully dissolved, then add the remaining water and stir again. Remove from the heat and leave to cool fully.

3. Prepare the beetroots by washing them and trimming off any damaged areas, but do not peel. Cut the beetroots into large pieces (4–6 chunks per beet) and place in a large, wide-mouthed, clean glass jar.

4. Add the cooled salt water to the jar, leaving a 1cm gap at the top. Cover the jar with a clean piece of cloth and secure it with an elastic band, then place the jar in a corner of the kitchen out of direct light and leave for about 2 weeks.

5. After this time, strain the kvass into clean glass bottles and keep refrigerated. You can eat the fermented beetroots – grate or slice them into a salad or roast them in the oven with sea salt and avocado oil.

FERMENTATION TIPS:
Fermenting doesn't have to be difficult or scary. Make sure all containers, utensils and preparation surfaces are very clean to avoid contamination by harmful bacteria.

   If a white film appears on top of the kvass during fermentation, gently remove it with a spoon and a cloth, wiping away any deposits left on the edges. This is a harmless yeast that won't harm you but it might spoil the taste of your kvass if left to develop, or worse, it could lead to mould growing. If your ferment develops signs of mould, throw it away, sterilise the jar and start again!

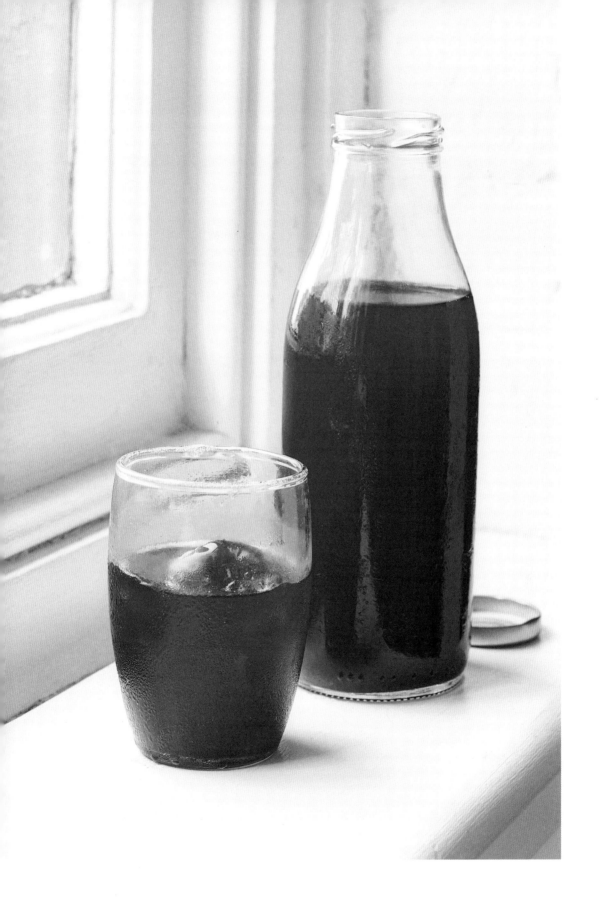

PMS protector

The liver is a vital organ for oestrogen clearance, which happens in two stages: the oestrogen is 'prepared' for clearance, then elimination is the second stage. Incorrect gut microbiome balance, low nutrient levels and poor fibre intake can impact the 'elimination' phase, and many key nutrients are needed for both stages of oestrogen clearance, including B vitamins, magnesium, zinc and selenium. Fibre is essential for 'getting things moving', as well as eliminating old oestrogen from the body and balancing hormones.

400ml unsweetened nut milk
1 ripe avocado, peeled and stoned
1 banana – the greener the better!
30ml kefir (coconut kefir is perfect)
1 tbsp golden linseeds
1 tbsp chia seeds
1 tbsp cacao powder, plus extra to serve
1 tbsp collagen peptides (optional)
1 tsp pumpkin seed butter
1 tbsp Brazil nut butter or 2 Brazil nuts,
    plus extra to chop and sprinkle on top
1 scoop Smooth Mag (optional – this powdered
    blend is rich in magnesium and B6, see page 97)

1. Add all the ingredients to the blender and combine on a high setting. Top with a sprinkle of cacao and chopped Brazil nuts.

Liver-loving latte

The delicious blend of spices and cacao in this latte is both comforting and helps to support liver function – essential for balanced hormones!

1 mug of unsweetened
    nut milk of choice
1 tsp cacao powder
½ tsp ground cinnamon
½ tsp ground turmeric
½ tsp ground ginger
1 tsp collagen
    peptides (optional)
Small amount of raw
    honey (optional)
A crack of black pepper

1. Warm the nut milk in a saucepan, then add all the remaining ingredients, except the pepper, and stir or whisk in until dissolved. Add a crack of black pepper and enjoy.

Stress recovery tonic

Our adrenal glands can take a pounding when we are under chronic stress ... this tonic provides the key nutrients needed to support these important organs.

30ml Beet kvass (store-bought or homemade, page 110)
20ml sea buckthorn juice (or lime juice, but ideally sea buckthorn!)
20ml raw apple cider vinegar
Sparkling water, to top up

TO SERVE
Fresh mint leaves, or add a few sprigs of mint into your ice-cube tray to make minty ice
A few pomegranate seeds

1. Add each ingredient to a tall glass and stir until combined. Add fresh mint or minty ice cubes and a few pomegranate seeds for extra goodness.

Beauty & the beet tonic

This tonic has all the makings of a happy gut and happy skin. Packed with antioxidants, probiotics and vitamin C, this daily dose of goodness will bring out your inner goddess.

30ml Beet kvass (store-bought or homemade, page 110)
30ml kombucha (when buying kombucha, look for low-sugar options, see page 78)
Juice of 1 lime
Sparkling water, to top up

TO SERVE
Ice cubes
A sprig of fresh mint, or add a few sprigs of mint into your ice-cube tray to make minty ice

1. Add all the ingredients to a tall glass, topping with sparkling water, ice cubes and a few sprigs of mint.

Happy hormones hot chocolate

Rich and delicious – everything a hot chocolate should be. The more your palate adapts to a low-sugar lifestyle, the darker the chocolate you will tolerate. Try 80% cocoa solids buttons and above to start, working up to 90–95%.

1 mug of hazelnut milk or
   unsweetened nutmilk
   of choice
25g raw cacao buttons
   (90% cocoa solids)
10g collagen peptides (optional)
½ tsp mushroom powder
   – I use Lion's Mane

1. Warm the nut milk in a saucepan before adding the remaining ingredients and stirring to combine and to melt the chocolate buttons.

2. If need be, transfer the smooth hot chocolate to a suitable heatproof blender and run on high speed to froth it to a velvety texture.

VARIATION
For a variation, use mint-chocolate buttons or chocolate orange, just make sure to keep the sugar low.

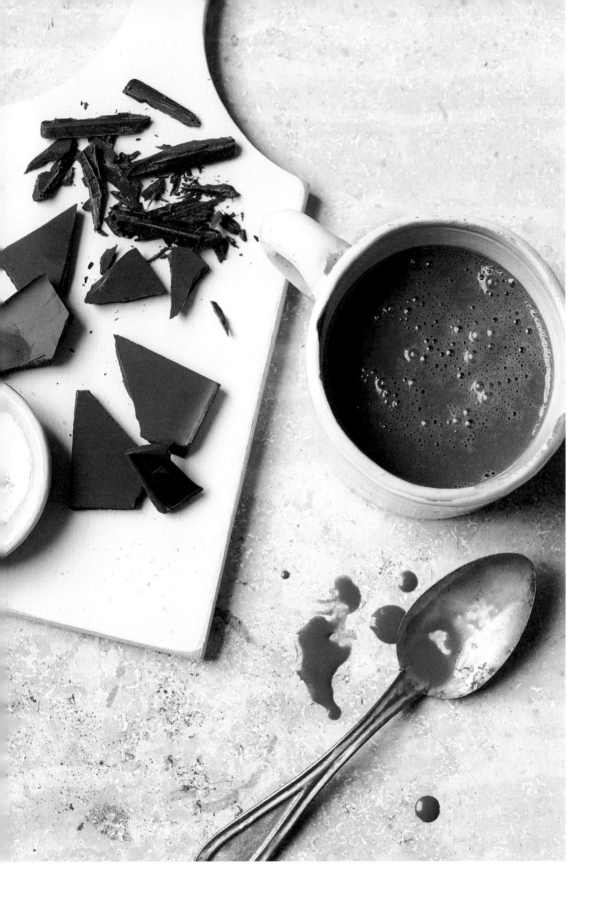

Allergy-tea

The perimenopause can be a time when allergies go into overdrive – runny, stuffy nose, itchy skin and migraines. Stinging nettles may offer some relief here. While research on the anti-histamine effects of stinging nettles is far from conclusive, these greens also offer a great range of nutrients, such as iron, magnesium, potassium and zinc, making this tea a top choice. The green tea included here is rich in a compound called quercetin, a natural anti-histamine, which will help alleviate allergy symptoms.

A large handful of carefully
    picked stinging nettles
    (pick using gloves!)
I green tea bag
I small lemon wedge
A slice of fresh ginger

1. Carefully wash the stinging nettle stems and, wearing gloves, snip off some of the leaves.

2. Boil the kettle and steep the nettle leaves in a mug of hot water for 5 minutes, then strain out the leaves and transfer the liquid to a clean mug.

3. Add the green tea bag, lemon wedge and ginger slice to the hot nettle water, stir and leave to steep for a minute or two, then drink while hot.

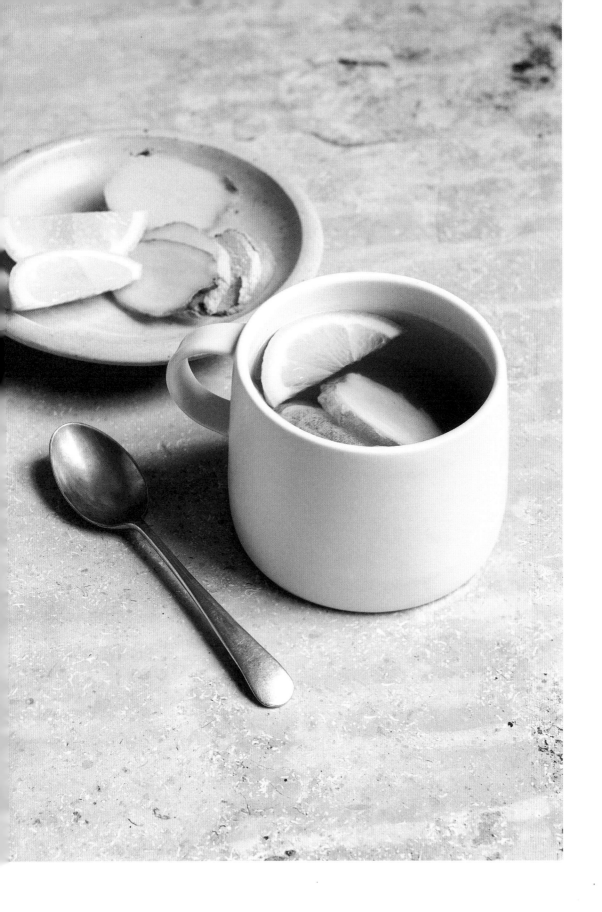

Hot flush tonic

While not all the properties of sage have been extensively researched, some studies indicate that it could be helpful for menopausal symptoms such as hot flushes. However, sage also has a chemical compound that, when taken in large quantities or for too long a period, could cause adverse side-effects such as headaches and vomiting. If you are taking any medication for blood pressure or diabetes, or are undergoing cancer treatment, consult your doctor before regularly consuming sage tea. Sage is generally considered safe when used in food recipes, but be cautious when taking it as supplemental capsules or oral essential oils.

5–6 fresh sage leaves
or 1 tsp dried sage
1 lemon wedge

1. Boil a kettle of water and set the leaves and lemon wedge in a heatproof mug. Pour over the boiled water, then set to one side to infuse and cool.

2. When ready to drink, remove the leaves and lemon wedge and take the cooled liquid to bed. Sip on the tonic before bed and again during the night if you find yourself awake and experiencing night sweats or hot flushes.

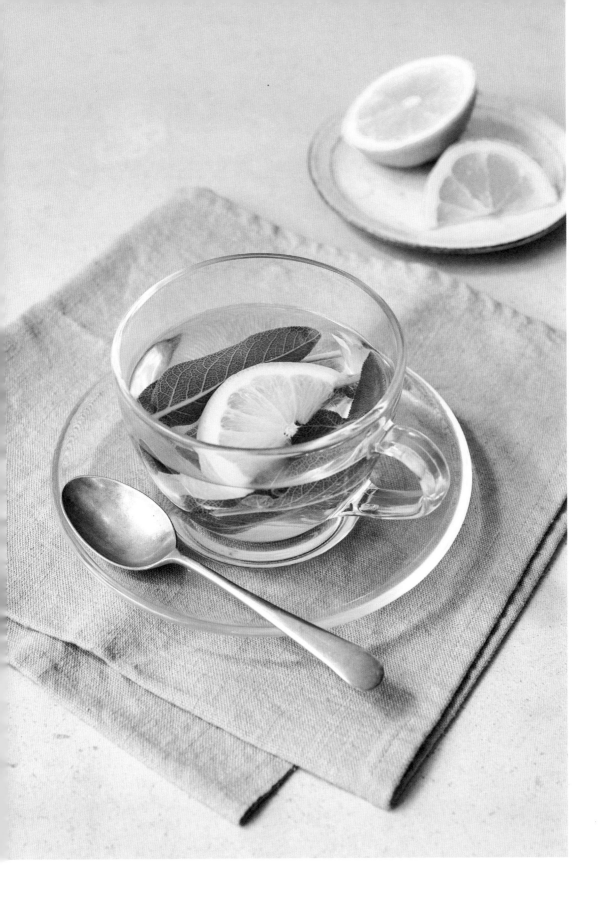

Feeling fruity (for libido & sexual energy)

This smoothie isn't hugely sweet, however, persevere and in time your palate will adapt and become accustomed to less sugar! Some of the ingredients on this list are a little quirky, such as Orange Burst, which is rich in omega-7 and good for reducing internal dryness and increasing lubrication, and Cordyceps mushroom powder, which is known as the Himalayan Viagra because it has aphrodisiac properties. If you don't have all of these ingredients, that's OK, just leave them out. Below is the complete list, but do pick and choose as you feel fit … and get fruity!

400ml unsweetened nut milk of choice
A handful of frozen mixed berries (blueberries, raspberries, blackcurrants)
1 ripe avocado, peeled and stoned
1 tsp tahini paste (black is super high in antioxidants)
1 tbsp chia seeds
1 tbsp collagen peptides
1 tsp Orange Burst (see page 97)
1 tsp Cordyceps mushroom powder

TO SERVE
Pumpkin seeds and sesame seeds, for sprinkling

1. Add all the ingredients except the seeds to a blender and combine until smooth.

2. Top with a sprinkle of pumpkin seeds and sesame seeds before serving.

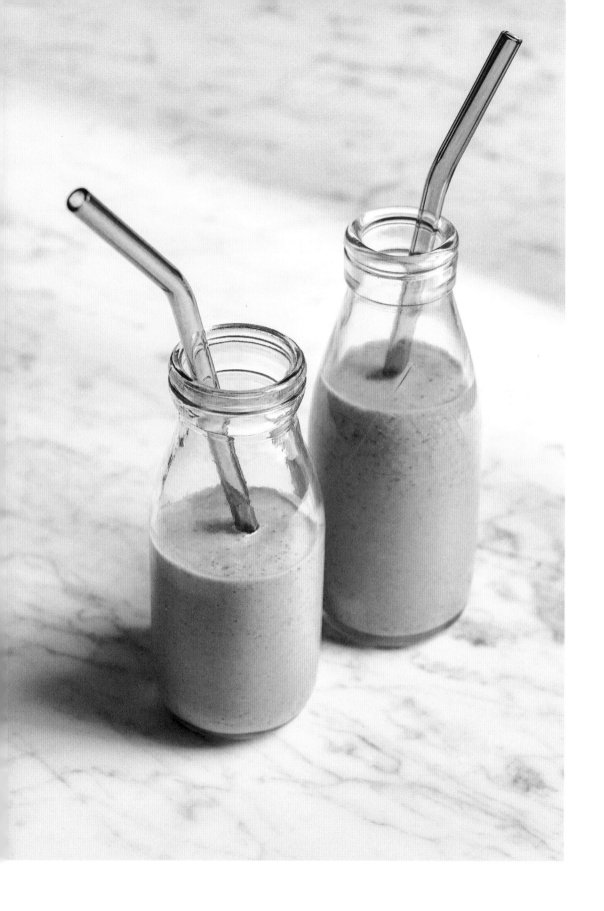

Red velvet

Nitrate-rich foods such as beetroot are incredibly important for building nitric oxide, a key compound for increasing blood flow to the skin, vagina and pelvic organs, which optimises cardiovascular health, mental clarity, healing and recovery from injury.

5–6 wedges of cold,
    roasted beetroot
A handful of frozen raspberries
2 tbsp cacao powder
400ml unsweetened nut milk
1 tsp mushroom powder – I use Lion's
    Mane (optional)
1 tbsp collagen peptides
    (optional)
1 tbsp maca powder (optional)

TO SERVE
Seeds and crushed nuts
    of choice

1. Add all the ingredients to a blender and combine until smooth. Finish with some seeds and crushed nuts of choice on top (pecans work well!).

(Photographed opposite)

Get a move along

When our hormones shift, things can get a little stuck in the bowel department. Keeping regular is essential for hormonal balance and bowel health. This smoothie will help move things along! Start with ½ teaspoon of the MCT oil – it has a powerful laxative effect.

400ml unsweetened nut milk
A handful of frozen blueberries
1 ripe avocado, peeled and stoned
1 tbsp collagen peptides
Juice of 1 lime
1 tbsp chia seeds
1 tbsp golden linseeds
½–1 tsp of MCT oil (see page 82)
1 fermented milk thistle capsule (optional,
    but super effective! See page 99)

OPTIONAL EXTRAS
Raw honey
A handful of Grain-no-la (see page 133)

1. Add all the ingredients to the blender and combine until smooth. This is not a sweet smoothie, it's zingy and packed with antioxidants, so add a touch of raw honey, if needed, and top with a handful of Grain-no-la for extra texture and flavour, if you like.

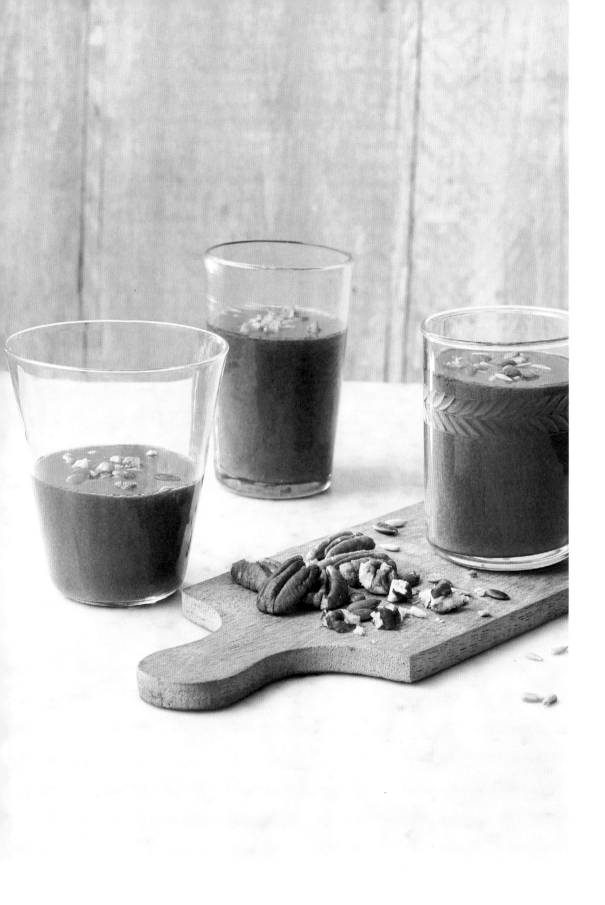

Energising smoothie

This energising, liver-loving, hormone-balancing, fibre-packed smoothie will give you a spring in your step! You can double up on the quantities and pour this into ice-lolly moulds, then freeze to make a healthy frozen dessert, too.

400ml unsweetened nut milk
100g frozen cauliflower
     rice (homemade, see page 143,
     or store-bought)
2 small carrots, roughly chopped
1 small apple, cored
     and roughly chopped
1 tsp ground cinnamon, plus extra to serve
½ tsp allspice
A handful of pecans
1 tbsp collagen peptides (optional)
1 tsp mushroom powder – I use Lion's Mane

1. Add all of the ingredients to a blender and combine until smooth. Finish with a sprinkle of cinnamon.

(Photographed opposite)

Skin saviour smoothie

Providing the body with key ingredients, including vitamins C and E, zinc and omega-7, is essential for healthy, elastic and bright skin. Our body also needs vitamin C in order to build collagen, the structural support of our skin, and sea buckthorn provides a super hit of this and omega-7. The boost of anti-ageing antioxidants from tahini can also reduce free-radical damage and slow premature ageing.

400ml unsweetened nut milk
1 ripe avocado, peeled and stoned
A handful of frozen or fresh berries
20ml sea buckthorn juice or
     1 tbsp sea buckthorn powder
1 tbsp sunflower seeds
1 tsp pumpkin seeds
1 tsp black tahini paste
1 tbsp chia seeds, plus extra for topping
1 tbsp collagen peptides
1 fermented milk thistle capsule (optional,
     liver and gut health is essential for skin health!
     See page 99)

1. Add all the ingredients to a blender and combine until smooth and creamy. Top with a sprinkle of chia seeds.

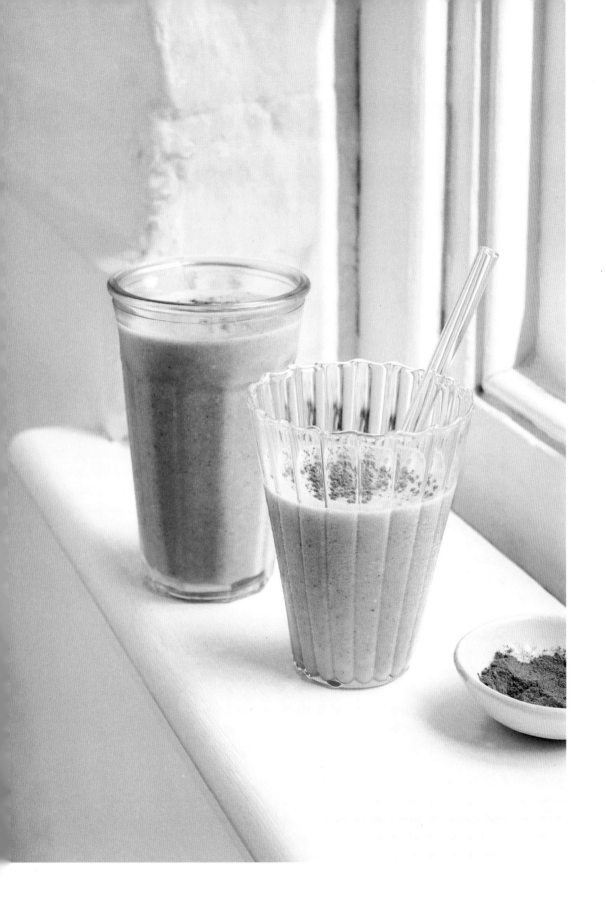

Keep calm &
carry on smoothie

This smoothie has key nutrients to help calm and soothe the nervous system. Packing in a nutrient-dense smoothie to support the nervous system is a great way to start the day. Intelligent fats, EPA, zinc, magnesium, B6 and probiotics all help to support happy brain chemistry and brain function. Fermented rhodiola is known for its abilities to promote harmony and resilience, and is used as a traditional remedy to fight depression, anxiety and fatigue.

400ml unsweetened nut milk of choice
1 ripe avocado, peeled and stoned
1 banana
1 tbsp unsweetened nut butter
1 tbsp tahini paste
1 tsp pumpkin seed butter
1 tsp CatchFree Omega – Tropical Mango (optional, vegan source of omega-3 EPA, see page 95)
1 fermented rhodiola capsule (optional)
A handful of chopped pecans, to serve

1. Add all the ingredients to a blender and combine until smooth. Top with a handful of chopped pecans.

Cavegirl

For a big hit of nutrient-dense ingredients … not your run-of the-mill smoothie! For those who are not fans of liver, heart and kidney but want all the benefits, organ meat capsules offer a full spectrum of nutrients.

400ml unsweetened nut milk
1 ripe avocado, peeled and stoned
1 banana or a handful of frozen berries
2 tbsp cacao powder
1 tsp collagen peptides
1 tsp black tahini paste
1 tsp mushroom powder – I use Lion's Mane
A pinch of salt
3 organ meat capsules (optional)

1. Add all of the ingredients to a blender and combine until smooth.

Breakfasts

Super simple crepe

With three ingredients, and taking just two minutes to make, these protein-packed crepes will soon become your number one speedy breakfast. They make a delicious and healthy start to the day or a great lunchtime alternative to a sandwich.

1 egg
A splash of unsweetened
    nut milk
A pinch of salt
Coconut oil or ghee, for frying

1. Beat the egg, nut milk and salt together in a bowl to create your batter.

2. Heat a standard-sized frying pan and melt the fat before adding all the batter, to cover the base of the whole frying pan.

3. Cook for 1 minute before carefully flipping over to cook for a further minute on the other side.

FILLING IDEAS
Whipped Roquefort (page 162), rocket and cucumber, goats' cheese and Raw slaw (page 154) with mixed leaves, grated green apple, feta and pea shoots, garlic mushrooms and crème fraîche … Fruity, savoury or a mixture of both, the possibilities are endless!

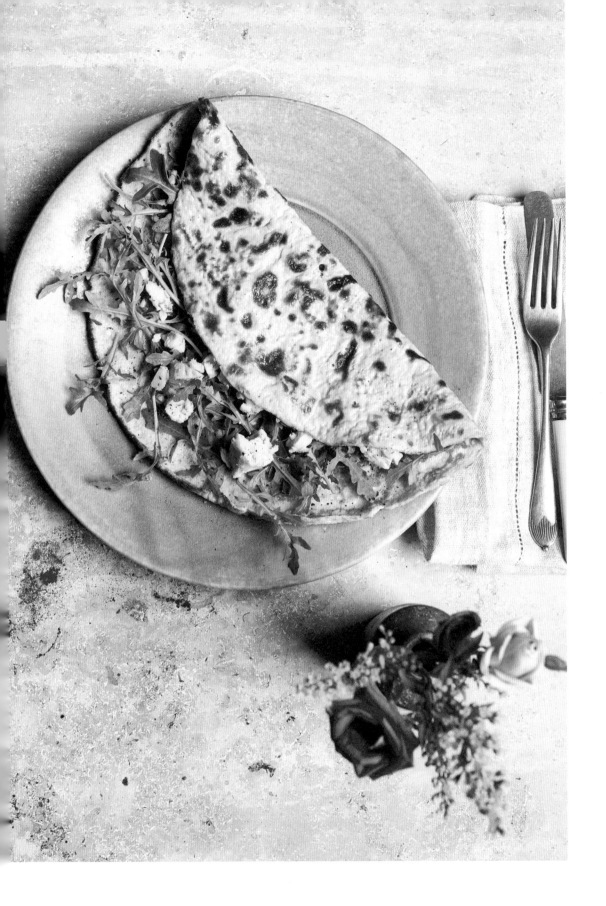

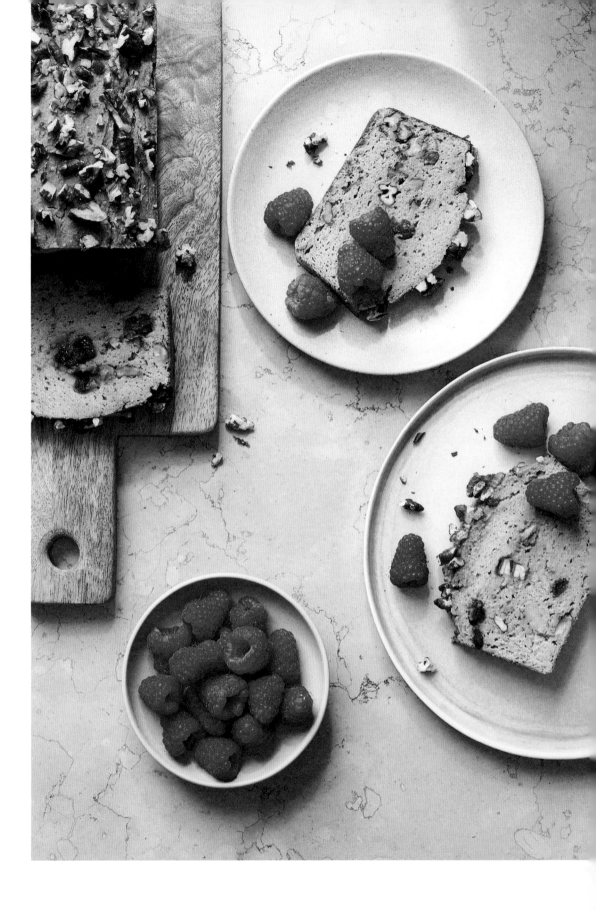

Banana & crunchy pecan loaf

This super simple banana loaf takes minutes to prepare and is packed with protein. A low-sugar version of the classic banana bread means good news for your blood sugars! Make a loaf and keep in the fridge – not least because there are two further recipes using this super simple loaf on page 245.

1. Preheat the oven to 180°C fan and line a 450g loaf tin with parchment paper (or the loaf tin liner inserts you can buy are super handy!).

2. Add all of the ingredients, except the pecans and sultanas, if using, to a blender and combine until thick and smooth. Add the sultanas, if using, and half of the chopped pecans to the mixture.

3. Pour the mixture into your lined loaf tin and top with the remaining pecans. Bake for 30–35 minutes until spongy to the touch. Allow to cool before slicing.

This breakfast loaf isn't particularly sweet, it's a low-sugar option that works well served with a dollop of natural or coconut yoghurt, a handful of raspberries or a spoonful of Blueberry and lime chia jam (see page 134) and a few extra nuts.

6 eggs
100g ground almonds
50g coconut flour
50ml unsweetened
    nut milk
1 ripe avocado, peeled
    and stoned
2 bananas
3 tsp ground cinnamon
1 tsp salt
A generous handful
    of pecans, or your
    favourite nuts
A handful of sultanas
    (optional)

BREAKFASTS

131

Mashed salted-avo delight

Salted, mashed avocados and warm toasted seedy bread are a match made in low-carb heaven. For low-carb bread and roll options, see Bread + Buns section, page 169.

2 Best buns (see page 170)
    or 4 slices of low-carb loaf
2 ripe avocados, peeled
    and stoned
Juice of 1 lime
1 small red onion, finely chopped
Small knob of butter
Sprinkle of chopped
    fresh coriander
Beetroot salt

1. Heat the grill. Slice the buns through the centre into three equally thick pieces and place under the grill, or place the loaf slices under the grill. Toast on both sides.

2. Place the avocado flesh into a bowl and roughly mash, adding the lime juice and finely chopped red onion.

3. Butter the toasted bread or buns, then spread with the mashed avocado and sprinkle over the coriander and beetroot salt.

VARIATIONS
Try adding smoked salmon, a chopped red onion and tomato salsa or egg mayonnaise with rocket.

Apple & cinnamon grain-no-la

A nutritious, fibre-packed, low-carb granola alternative that will keep your blood sugars stable and your belly feeling full!

1. Preheat the oven to 170°C fan.

2. Core and chop the apples into chunks, add to a blender or food processor and blend to a purée.

3. Place half of all of the remaining ingredients in a mixing bowl.

4. Place the other half of the remaining ingredients into the blender or food processor with the puréed apple and combine. Once well combined, transfer to the mixing bowl with the reserved ingredients. Mix well.

5. Line a baking tray with parchment paper before transferring clumps of the nutty-seed mix, then spreading it evenly over the tray.

6. Bake for 20 minutes. Remove from the oven and allow to cool on the tray. Store in a glass, sealed jar or airtight container for up to 7 days.

Add in a few sultanas for a touch of extra sweetness, if desired.

2 apples
100g almonds
100g shredded coconut
100g golden linseeds
50g coconut oil, melted
50g sesame seeds
50g sunflower seeds
50g pecans
50g chia seeds
25g Brazil nuts
40g maple syrup
3 tsp ground cinnamon
1½ tsp salt

BREAKFASTS

N-oatmeal with natural yoghurt & blueberry & lime chia jam

A calcium-rich, liver-loving start to the morning that will leave you feeling energised and ready to tackle the day ahead!

350ml full-fat coconut milk
or unsweetened nut milk
4 tbsp shelled hemp seeds
or hearts
4 tbsp ground almonds
2 tbsp desiccated coconut
I tbsp collagen peptides
(optional)
3 tbsp chia seeds
I tsp ground cinnamon
I–2 tsp erythritol or maple
syrup (optional)

BLUEBERRY AND LIME CHIA JAM
125g punnet of blueberries
Juice of I unwaxed lime
I generous tbsp chia seeds

TO SERVE
Natural or coconut yoghurt
Zest of I unwaxed lime
A few chopped nuts

1. Add the milk to a pan and gently heat it through on a medium heat.

2. Add all the other ingredients to the warmed milk, turn down the heat to a lower setting and leave to thicken for 5–8 minutes, stirring occasionally.

3. In a separate pan, add the blueberries and lime juice and gently heat until the blueberries break down to a jammy consistency. Add the chia seeds and combine well, allowing to cool and thicken.

4. Transfer the prepared n-oatmeal to two bowls, top with a dollop of yoghurt and of the blueberry and lime chia jam, then sprinkle with the lime zest and a few chopped nuts.

If you make enough for two but only eat one, you can use the mixture to make a delicious tray of N-oat bars (see page 242).

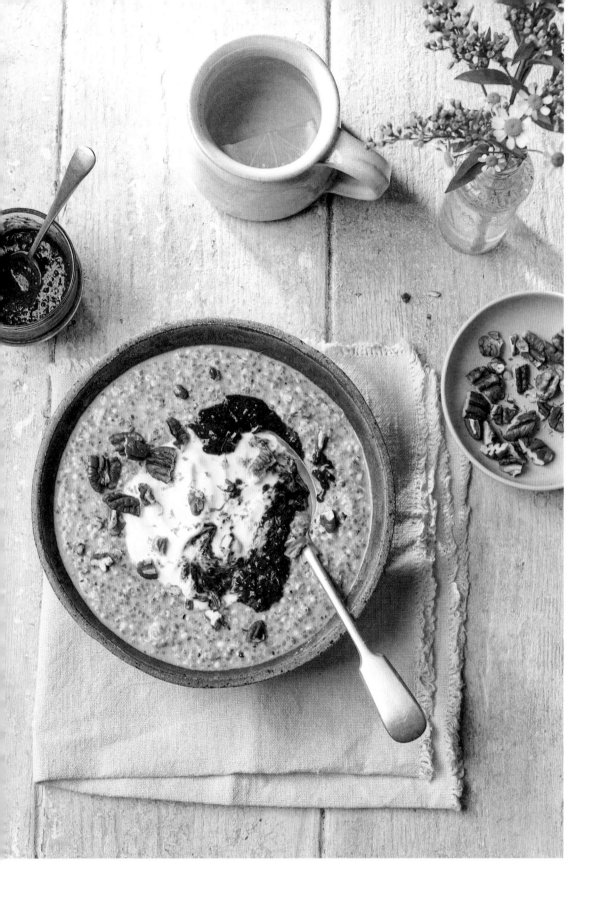

Apple-spiced n-oatmeal with natural yoghurt & pecans

A warm and comforting low-carb version of porridge oats, packed with fibre and bursting with nutrients. Get your day started with a burst of energy!

Coconut oil or butter,
  for frying
2 apples, cored and
  cut into cubes
1 tsp miso paste
2 tsp ground cinnamon,
  plus extra to serve
350–400ml full-fat coconut milk
  or unsweetened nut milk
4 tbsp shelled hemp seeds
  or hearts
4 tbsp ground almonds
2 tbsp desiccated coconut
1 tbsp collagen peptides
  (optional)
2 tbsp chia seeds
½ tsp salt
1–2 tsp erythritol, maple syrup
  or raw honey (optional)

TO SERVE
A dollop of coconut or natural
  yoghurt, to serve
A handful of chopped pecans

1. Add a little coconut oil or butter to a saucepan and gently fry the cubed apple, miso and cinnamon for 6–8 minutes until slightly softened. Pour the nut milk or coconut milk into the saucepan and warm along with the softened apple.

2. Add all the other ingredients to the warmed nut milk and apple and stir for 5–6 minutes until it begins to thicken.

3. Transfer the n-oatmeal to two bowls, top each with a dollop of yoghurt, a small handful of chopped pecans and a sprinkling of cinnamon.

For an alternative, add cacao powder, stirring in fresh raspberries once the n-oatmeal is made.

The taste of paradise – coconut & pecan pancakes

These fibre-packed pancakes have a rich, buttery sweetness from the pecan pieces, combined with a tangy hit of blueberry from the chia jam topping.

4 large eggs
30g chopped pecans
2 tbsp coconut flour
1 tbsp ground almonds
1 tsp ground cinnamon
½ tsp salt
½ tsp baking powder
50ml unsweetened nut milk
Coconut oil, for frying
Blueberry and lime chia jam,
    to serve (see page 134)

1. Beat the eggs and add the chopped pecans, coconut flour, ground almonds, cinnamon, salt, baking powder and nut milk. The batter will be runny!

2. Heat a large frying pan and add a dollop of coconut oil. Add a serving spoon of batter to the pan (they will not be perfect circles), using the batter in batches. Allow the pancakes to form and lightly brown for 2–3 minutes before flipping, then cooking for a further 2–3 minutes. Keep warm while you cook the remaining pancakes.

3. Serve with a dollop of Blueberry and lime chia jam.

VARIATIONS
Omit the cinnamon and add some finely chopped red onion instead of pecans, and top with sour cream and smoked salmon, or mashed avocados, tomatoes and salt for a vegetarian alternative.

BREAKFASTS

Green banana get up & go pancakes

These protein-packed, flourless pancakes can be made without the collagen, however, the extra hit of amino acids in the morning is ideal for muscle building and hunger control. When bananas are green, they have less sugar content … you decide how green you want to go. Delicious hot or cold!

1 greenish banana
2 eggs
1 tbsp collagen peptides
  (optional)
½ tsp ground cinnamon
Coconut oil or ghee, for frying

TO SERVE
Natural yoghurt, fresh
  berries, chopped nuts
  and seeds

1. Add the banana to a blender with the eggs, collagen (if using) and cinnamon, then combine to create a smooth batter.

2. Heat a small amount of coconut oil or ghee in a frying pan, and when the pan is hot, add 3–4 spoons of batter to create 3–4 mini pancakes. Cook for 2–4 minutes until golden in colour before flipping over to cook on the other side.

3. Serve with natural yoghurt, fresh berries, chopped nuts and seeds for extra goodness.

BREAKFASTS

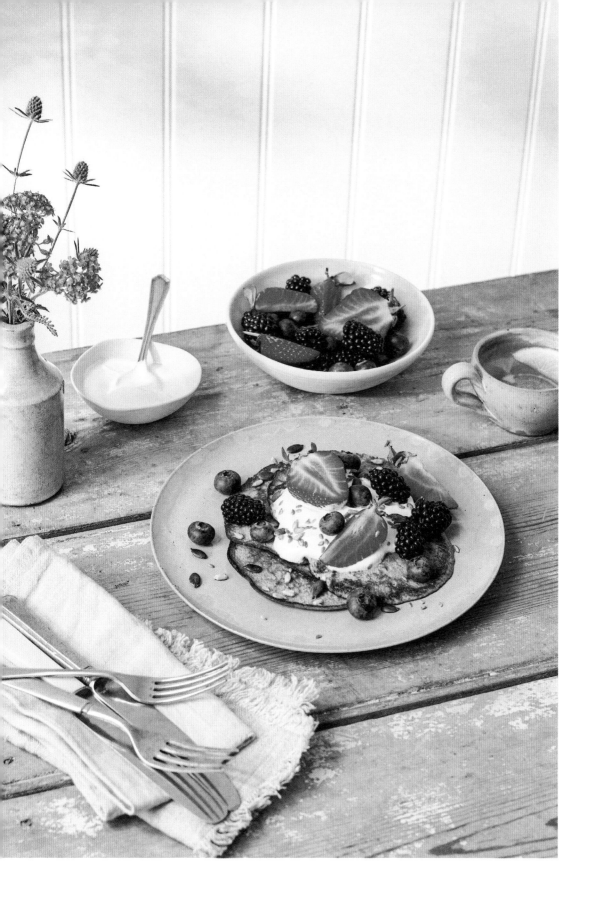

Blender breakfast loaf – smoked salmon & salted pistachio loaf

This is the ultimate in fast-food baking; a protein-packed loaf that can be eaten for breakfast, brunch or lunch.

6 eggs
100g ground almonds
100ml melted butter,
    ghee or coconut oil
1 ripe avocado, peeled
    and stoned
4 tbsp nutritional yeast
1 tsp salt
1 tsp baking powder
100g smoked salmon
A handful of shelled pistachios
    or nuts of choice
A pinch of coarse sea salt

1. Preheat the oven to 180°C fan and line a 450g loaf tin with parchment paper (or the loaf tin liner inserts you can buy are super handy!).

2. Add all of the ingredients except the salmon, nuts and salt to a blender and combine until thick and smooth.

3. Next add the salmon to the blender and pulse to roughly combine.

4. Pour the mixture into your lined loaf tin and top with a handful of pistachio nuts, then sprinkle with coarse sea salt.

5. Bake for 30–35 minutes until spongy to the touch. Allow to cool before slicing. Delicious hot or cold.

ALTERNATIVE
Substitute salmon with flaked haddock or feta chunks as a tasty alternative.

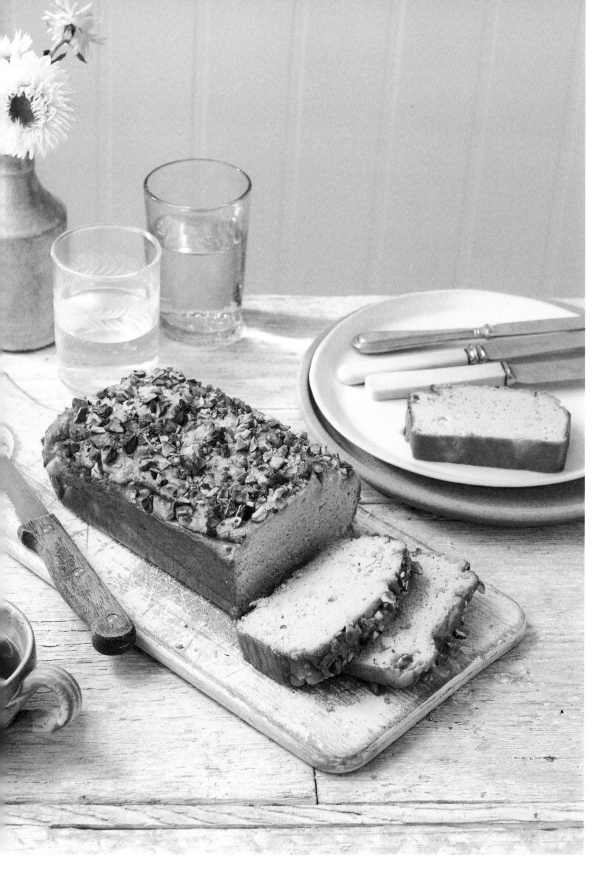

Sides + Dressings

Cauliflower rice three ways

Cauliflower rice tastes SO much better than you may think – fluffy and flavoursome, it has a fraction of the carbs of regular rice and is packed with fibre and nutrients. It makes the perfect carrier for curries and a wonderful base for many an easy meal. Having a packet of store-bought cauli-rice in the cupboard can be a saviour when you need a meal in minutes. FullGreen make an ambient riced cauliflower product, widely available in most supermarkets. However, making your own cauli-rice is also super simple and it can be used in a whole variety of ways!

Allow ½ cauliflower per serving

Plain cauli rice

2–3 large heads of cauliflower

1. Preheat the oven to 160–170°C fan.

2. Remove the outer leaves of the cauliflower, cutting it into florets. Add 6–7 florets to a food processor and pulse (not pulverise!) to a couscous consistency.

3. Place a layer (about 5cm thick) of raw cauli rice onto a baking tray, using multiple trays to batch cook. Bake for 5–6 minutes, remove from the oven and stir before returning to the oven, cooking for a further 5–6 minutes.

Keep in the fridge for up to 3 days. Alternatively freeze the cauliflower after you have riced it (before cooking) and take it out to defrost, then cook before using in the recipes on the next page.

Moroccan cauli rice with spring onions

500g cooked cauli-rice
  (see page 143)
I tsp ras-el-hanout
4 spring onions, chopped
40g chopped fresh coriander
  (stalks removed)
50g toasted cashews
  (place the cashews in an oven
  at 180°C fan for 5–6 minutes)
A handful of pumpkin seeds
½ tsp salt and black pepper,
  to taste

1. As the cauli rice cools, add all the ingredients and mix in evenly.

2. Keep in the fridge for up to 3 days.

Turmeric & coconut cauli rice

500g cooked cauli-rice
  (see page 143)
I tsp turmeric
80g desiccated coconut
50g toasted cashews
  (place the cashews in an oven
  at 180°C fan for 5–6 minutes)
A handful of sunflower seeds
A handful of chopped
  spring onions
½ tsp salt and black pepper,
  to taste

1. As the cauli rice cools, add all the ingredients and mix in evenly.

2. Keep in the fridge for up to 3 days.

3. Add variations such as pomegranate seeds, fresh mint leaves, chopped olives, fresh basil and sundried tomatoes. The flavour combinations really are endless!

(Photographed opposite)

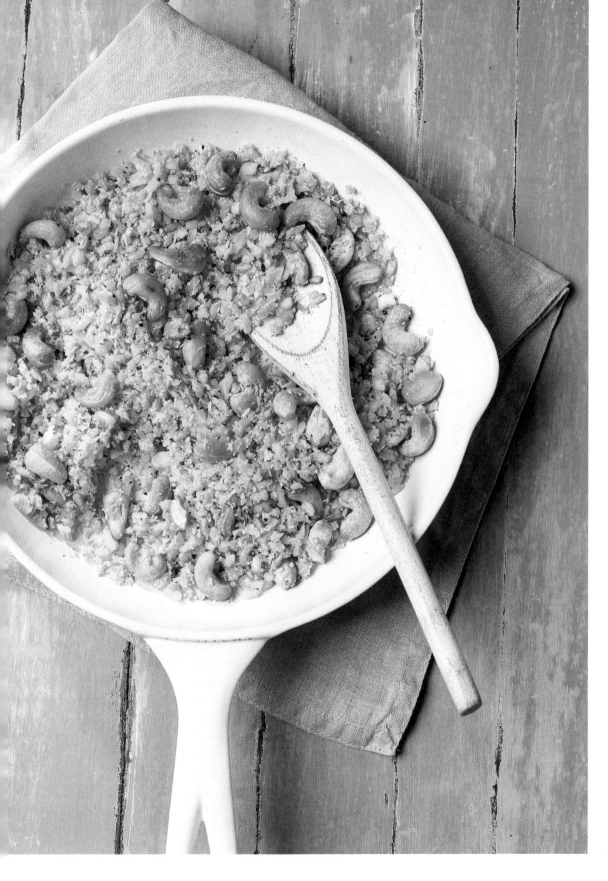

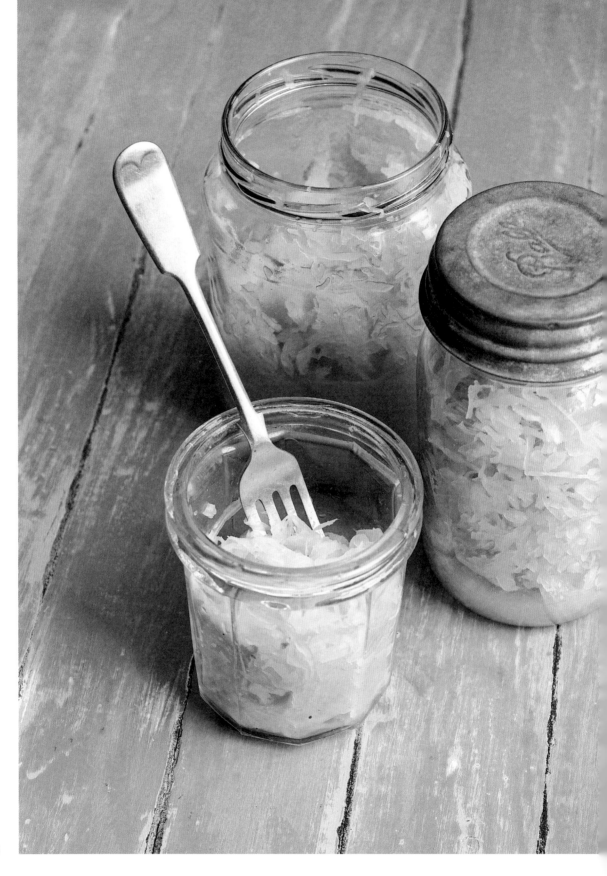

Speedy sauerkraut

Sauerkraut is the ultimate healthy food for the gut. Rich in probiotics, pre-digested cabbage (sexy, eh?!) and vitamin C, dolloping a daily dose of sauerkraut onto your plate is a simple way of upgrading any meal.

1. Before you start, make sure all your containers, utensils and preparation surfaces are very clean, to avoid contamination from unfriendly bacteria.

2. Make the brine: boil ½ litre of water in a saucepan and add the salt. Stir until fully dissolved, then add the rest of the water. Leave to cool fully.

3. Prepare the cabbage: don't wash it, the bacteria on the surface will start the fermentation process. Remove the first leaf and set aside. Trim the cabbage of any damaged areas. Slice the cabbage finely (a mandolin will give you the most consistent results, a sharp knife works just as well, or use the shredding blade on a food processor).

4. Place the cabbage in a large, clean wide-mouthed glass jar (Kilner-style with a rubber seal is ideal, but any jam jar is fine), and pack it in tightly, placing the outer cabbage leaf on top to act as a stopper, then cover with the cooled brine. The cabbage should be fully submerged, leaving 1cm clear at the top of the jar to allow for bubbles. (If you don't have enough brine, make another litre. You can keep the rest in the fridge for your next batch.)

5. Cover the jar with a lid, then place it in a corner of the kitchen with a plate or tray underneath, as it often leaks during the early stages of fermentation.

6. Bubbles will start forming after about 3–4 days. Once the bubbles die down, after about a week, the cabbage is fermented and you can start to eat it. If you are new to sauerkraut, have any bloating or digestive issues, eat an 'early fermentation', 2–3 days old. Otherwise, leaving it for up to 3 weeks increases the probiotic levels.

1 litre filtered water
40g fine Himalayan pink salt
1 small head of white or red cabbage (ideally organic)

FLAVOURING OPTIONS
This sauerkraut is delicious as it is, or you can add some extras for a different flavour. Here are some tasty variations:

— 1 tsp spice, such as cumin or fennel seeds, crushed juniper berries, pink peppercorns or nigella seeds

— A handful of fresh herbs, such as dill, wild garlic, thyme, oregano …

— A few slices of fresh ginger or turmeric root, 1 tbsp of grated horseradish or a couple of bashed garlic cloves

— A handful of dried seaweed

— A grated carrot or beetroot

SIDES + DRESSINGS

Raspberry blush vinaigrette

This salad dressing is delicious on grilled goat's cheese, steak or to liven up any salad! Full of antioxidants and vitamin C (for building progesterone), it's worth making a batch and having it to hand in the fridge.

100g raspberries
  (10–12 juicy raspberries)
60ml extra virgin olive oil
Juice of 1 lime
20ml balsamic vinegar
20ml Beet kvass (optional,
  but ideal, see page 110)
1 tsp salt (ideally beetroot salt)

1. Add all of the ingredients to a blender and combine. Transfer to a clean glass jar with a lid, keep in the fridge and use within 3 days.

Use with Grilled goat's cheese salad (page 208), Beetroot salted steak (page 198), Tickled pink pickled eggs (page 186) and Double beetroot salad (page 200).

SIDES + DRESSINGS

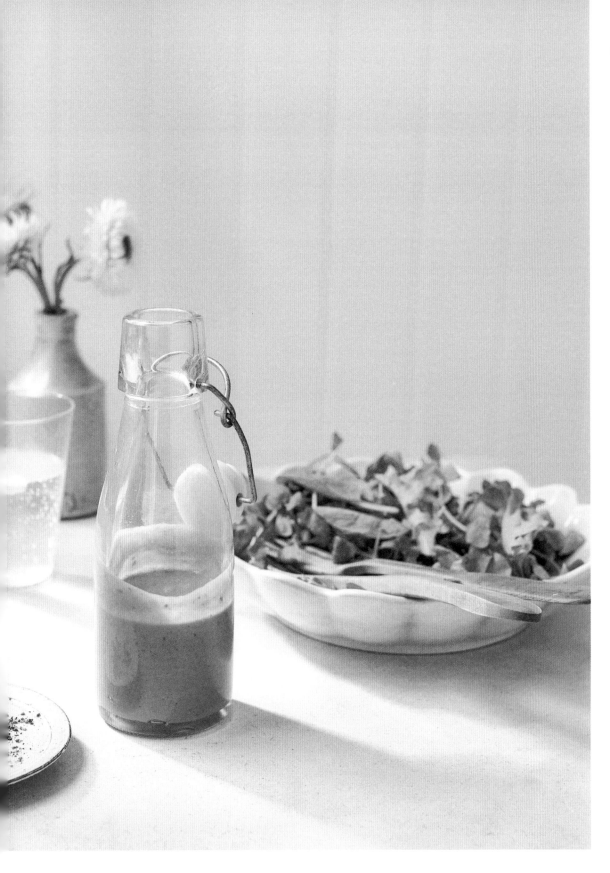

Black tahini & miso dressing

Black tahini is an *exceptionally* rich source of antioxidants; in traditional Chinese medicine, black sesame seeds are considered to be highly anti-ageing. It is also an excellent source of magnesium and calcium.

I tbsp black sesame
  tahini paste
4 tbsp extra virgin olive oil
I tbsp balsamic vinegar
I tbsp raw apple
  cider vinegar
I tsp miso paste
I tsp salt

1. Add the tahini, olive oil, both vinegars, miso and salt to a bowl and whisk together with a fork until combined.

2. Keep refrigerated and use within 5 days. It will thicken slightly in the fridge, so mix it up with a fork, loosen with a little olive oil or keep at room temperature for 30 minutes before serving.

Use on Roquefort, rocket and pink grapefruit salad (page 180), Kale, feta, walnut & pomegranate salad (page 194) and Broccoli & walnut whip (page 160).

SIDES + DRESSINGS

Lemon olive oil mayonnaise

Mayonnaise made with healthy fats is a fabulous, versatile fridge essential. Olive oil is made up of almost 75% anti-inflammatory, monounsaturated fats and is loaded with antioxidants. This mayonnaise makes a superb addition to many recipes, including Remoulade (see page 154).

1. Add the egg yolks, lemon juice and salt to a stand mixer or whisk by hand. Slowly add the light olive oil (in small drops). The mix will start to thicken and resemble mayonnaise; as it does you can add the oil a little faster. Keep refrigerated for up to 1 week.

3 egg yolks (room temperature)
Juice of 1 lemon
A pinch of salt
250ml light olive oil

BALMY BALSAMIC LEMON MAYO
For a twist on the classic Lemon olive oil mayonnaise, add 20ml of balsamic vinegar to it.

SIDES + DRESSINGS

Roast red pepper pesto

Sunflower seeds are a rich source of skin-loving vitamin E, and combined with the goodness of garlic, basil and olive oil, this pesto works on so many levels!

1 red pepper
60ml olive oil
15ml apple cider vinegar
1 tsp salt
1 garlic clove
1 tsp miso paste
30g sunflower seeds
A handful of fresh basil leaves

1. Preheat the oven to 170°C fan.

2. Prepare the pepper by removing the inner seeds, then roughly chopping. Place on a baking tray, coat with the olive oil and toss to combine (if you like, you can roast extra peppers at the same time to accompany the meal).

3. Roast in the oven for 30–40 minutes.

4. Add the roasted peppers and all the remaining ingredients to a blender and combine to produce a thick, delicious pesto.

USE WITH
Smokey chicken drumsticks (page 192), Baked avocados (page 183), Creamy curried cauli steaks (page 184), Frittata (page 207) and Keto-friendly chicken (page 220).

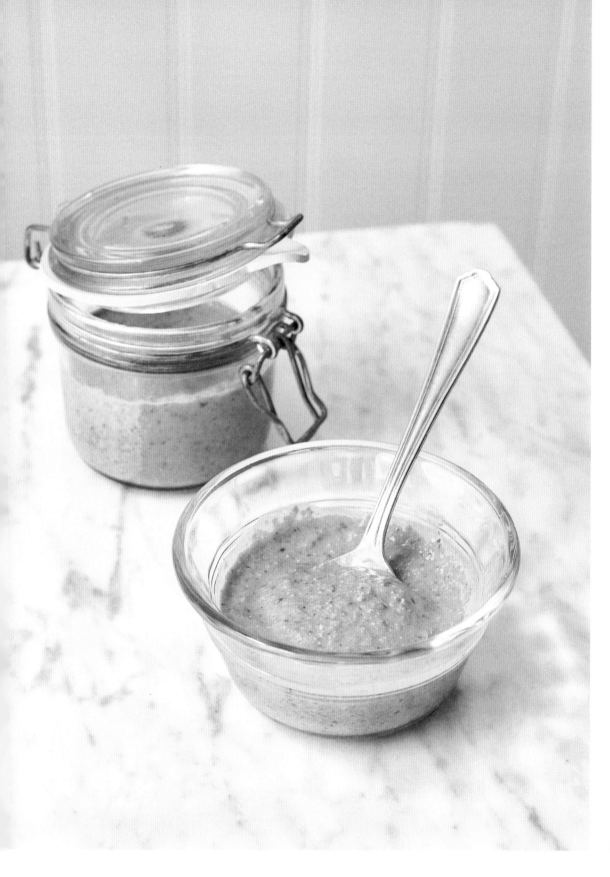

Celeriac three ways

Celeriac is a super versatile veggie. As well as being a powerhouse of nutrients, including our skin's best friend, vitamin C, it makes a great low-carb alternative to potato.

Remoulade

The perfect side dish – rich, creamy and deliciously healthy.

Serves 2–3

6 tbsp Lemon olive oil
   mayonnaise (see page 151)
2 tbsp Dijon mustard
1 tsp miso paste
A pinch of salt
1 small celeriac, peeled
   and quartered

1. In a mixing bowl, combine the mayonnaise, mustard, miso and salt.

2. Grate or shred the celeriac quarters in a food processor. Add the celeriac to the mayonnaise mix and stir until completely coated.

Serve this on toasted Low-carb loaf (page 174) with pea shoots or rocket.

Raw slaw

This rainbow of goodness will see your gut microbiome dancing for joy. Ideally choose organic vegetables if available.

Serves 2

1 beetroot
1 sweet potato
1 carrot
1 green apple
A handful of sunflower seeds
30ml olive oil
1 tbsp raw apple cider vinegar
1 tbsp balsamic vinegar
Beetroot salt or regular salt

1. Grate all of the veg, keeping the skin on for extra fibre, into a large mixing bowl.

2. Add the sunflower seeds and all remaining ingredients, then stir to combine and evenly coat the shredded veggies.

There is no end to the combination of veggies you could shred for raw slaw – try celeriac, cabbage, courgette. It's a great way of increasing your fibre for the day.

Dauphinoise

This low-carb version of the classic potato dauphinoise is comfort food at its best!

**Serves 2 as a main/
4 as a side dish**

1 medium-sized celeriac
80g Thai curry paste, or to taste,
depending on the brand
(R&G make superb pastes,
see page 83)
400ml tin of full-fat coconut milk

TO SERVE
Coconut yoghurt, a pinch of
salt and a sprinkle of fresh
coriander

1. Preheat the oven to 170°C fan.

2. Peel and quarter the celeriac before thinly slicing it using a sharp knife or a mandolin.

3. Add the curry paste and coconut milk to a saucepan and heat, stirring to combine. Add the celeriac slices and heat for a further 6–8 minutes, allowing the celeriac to start to soften (the sauce won't cover the whole of the celeriac, that's OK).

4. Scoop out the celeriac using a slotted spoon and transfer to an ovenproof dish before pouring over the Thai coconut sauce.

5. Bake in the oven for 30–40 minutes. Finish with a dollop of coconut yoghurt, a pinch of salt and a sprinkle of fresh coriander.

Serve as an accompaniment to a steak, or as a light meal with salad and sauerkraut.

Cauli-power cheese

All that cauli-goodness wrapped up in a cheese blanket. Alternatively, use broccoli or a combination of both.

1 medium-sized head
   of cauliflower
200g cream cheese
100ml double cream or
   unsweetened nut milk
½ tsp smoked paprika
70g grated Cheddar (keep
   a handful back for topping)
2 tbsp coconut aminos
A handful of chopped
   fresh herbs, to serve

1. Preheat the oven to 170°C fan.

2. Cut the cauliflower into florets and soften in a pan of gently boiling water for 6–8 minutes.

3. Add all the other ingredients to a blender and combine until a smooth sauce forms.

4. Drain the cooked cauliflower florets and combine in an ovenproof dish with the cheese sauce. Sprinkle with the reserved grated cheese and bake for 10–15 minutes. Remove and sprinkle with chopped fresh herbs.

SIDES + DRESSINGS

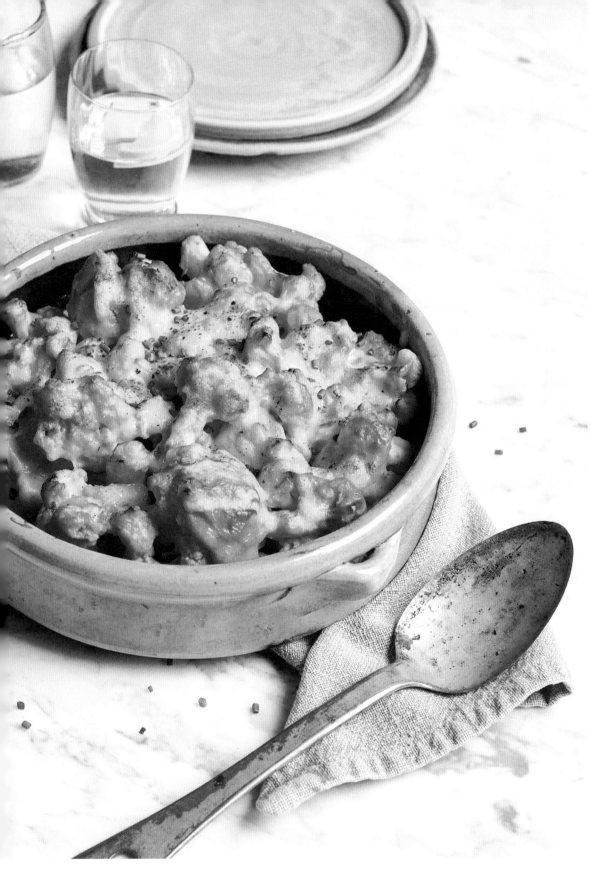

Easy-peasy liver pâté

Liver is one of the most nutrient-dense foods on the planet. Rich in vitamins A and B12, it is an inexpensive and delicious way to ramp up your nutrient levels!

300g liver (chicken is the mildest, but if you can find beef, it's delicious!)
1 tbsp apple cider vinegar
150g onions or shallots
300g ghee
Salt, black pepper, grated nutmeg and other spices of choice (chilli flakes, oregano, allspice, pink peppercorns)

1. Chop the liver into thumb-sized pieces, trimming off any discolouration and nerves as you go. Pat dry to remove excess blood and place in a bowl. Mix with the apple cider vinegar and leave to marinate while you dice the onions.

2. Melt 100g of the ghee in a pan and sauté the onions until softened. Add the liver and cook for approximately 5 minutes, until golden on the outside and still pink inside (much longer and the liver will become rubbery, resulting in grainy pâté). Remove from the heat and add seasoning.

3. Blend the contents of the pan in a food processor with 150g of the remaining ghee until smooth. Adjust the seasoning to taste, then spoon the pâté into a clean glass jar or two, avoiding any air bubbles.

4. Once the pâté has cooled, melt the remaining 50g of ghee, and pour over in a layer of approximately 4mm. Pop the lid on. Once sealed, this will keep for a week in the fridge. Once opened, store in the fridge and eat within 48 hours.

Serve with toasted, buttered Low-carb loaf (page 174).

SIDES + DRESSINGS

Golden beef bone broth

The perfect base for soups or as a warming drink, bone broth is brimming with goodness!
Bone broth is wonderfully nutritious, inexpensive and the ideal way to boost the nutrient content
of other meals when used in recipes.

1. Add all of the ingredients to a slow cooker or a large pan on the hob.
    Add enough water to cover the beef bones and cook at a low setting
    for 24–36 hours. Check occasionally, and if the water level becomes
    low, top up with extra water.

2. Strain the broth and allow to cool. Pour the strained stock into
    ice-cube trays and freeze (for up to 3 months) for easy-to-use bone
    broth cubes, or bottle up and keep in the fridge for up to 5 days.

TO MAKE GRAVY
Add 250ml (or desired amount of gravy base) to a pan and warm. Add
the warmed bone broth to a blender, add a heaped teaspoon of xanthan
gum and blend. The bone broth will instantly thicken, creating a rich,
unctuous gravy.

From your butcher, request
about 450g of beef bones,
including:
Chopped thigh bones
Marrow bone
Knuckle bone

1 large onion, unpeeled
   and roughly chopped
2 heads of garlic, unpeeled
4 celery stalks, unpeeled
   and chopped into quarters
4 medium carrots, chopped
   into quarters
2 tbsp garlic powder
1 tbsp ground turmeric
2 dried bay leaves
3 tbsp apple cider vinegar
2½ tsp Himalayan rock salt
Black pepper, to taste

SIDES + DRESSINGS

Broccoli & walnut whip

This delicious salad is a nutrient powerhouse. It takes minutes to whip up, with all that walnut goodness and broccoli brilliance leaving you full and satisfied.

I head of broccoli
I small red onion
A handful of walnuts
3 heaped tbsp natural
    or coconut yoghurt
4 tbsp Black tahini & miso
    dressing (page 150)
A handful of pomegranate seeds

1. Cut the broccoli into florets, and steam or gently boil them for 5 minutes until tender. Drain and rinse under cold water to prevent further cooking.

2. Dice the red onion and roughly chop most of the walnuts, leaving a few pieces to serve.

3. In a mixing bowl, combine the yoghurt and 3 tablespoons of the Black tahini & miso dressing.

4. Add the broccoli, red onion and walnuts to the mixing bowl with the yoghurt and stir to coat.

5. Plate up and finish with the remaining walnut pieces, drizzle over the remaining I tablespoon of the Black tahini & miso dressing and scatter over a few pomegranate seeds.

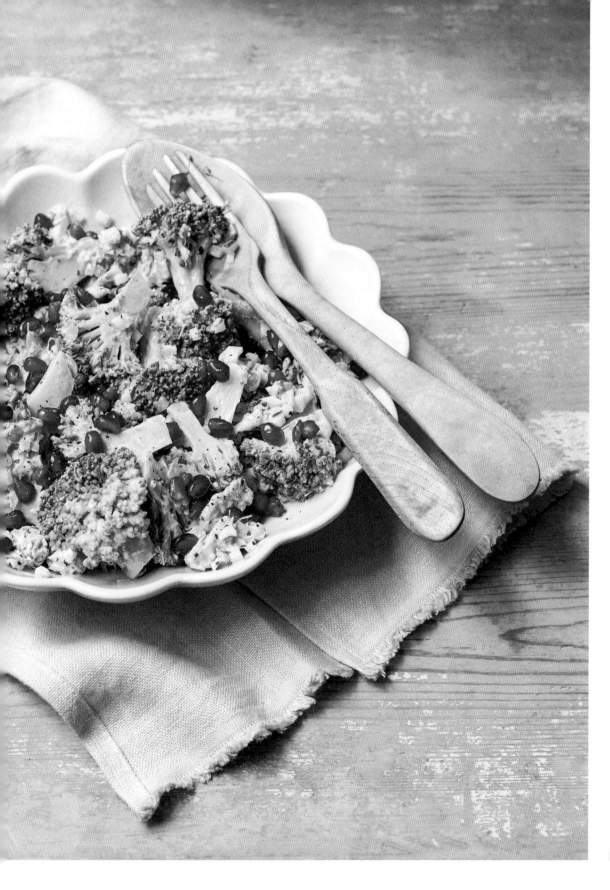

Whipped Roquefort & toasted thins

This is simply delicious … it takes minutes to make and is packed with gut-beneficial bacteria, fibre and protein. Roquefort is traditionally made from sheep's milk, which is easier to digest than cow's milk cheeses.

3–4 thin slices of Low-carb
    loaf (see page 174)
A good glug of olive oil
1 ripe avocado, peeled
    and stoned
100g Roquefort (ideally
    raw and unpasteurised)
1 small red onion
A handful of walnuts
Chopped fresh herbs of choice
    (chives work well)
A pinch of beetroot salt

1. Preheat the oven to 185°C fan. Place the thin slices of Low-carb loaf on a baking tray and coat both sides with olive oil.

2. Bake for 10–12 minutes, turning to brown both sides evenly.

3. In the meantime, add the avocado and Roquefort to a blender and whip until smooth and creamy, then transfer to a bowl.

4. Finely chop the red onion and add to the whipped cheese mix.

5. Roughly chop the walnuts and herbs.

6. Add the whipped Roquefort to the toasted thins and sprinkle with chopped walnuts, herbs and beetroot salt.

The whipped Roquefort also works well in Super simple crepes on page 128 or paired with simply roasted veggies such as cherry tomatoes, courgettes, onion, fennel and celery.

SIDES + DRESSINGS

Cauli-hummus with toasted sunflower seeds

This delicious, creamy cauliflower hummus is packed with antioxidants, fibre and healthy fats, keeping you fuller for longer and your blood sugars stable.

1. Preheat the oven to 170°C fan.

2. Break the cauliflower into florets and place them on a baking tray. Drizzle with 2 tablespoons of the olive oil and toss to combine. Roast in the oven for 25 minutes or until tender. Allow to cool for 10 minutes.

3. Add the sunflower seeds to a hot, dry pan and gently brown for a few minutes, watching closely to prevent them burning.

4. Add the cooled roasted cauliflower, tahini, remaining 2 tablespoons of olive oil, water, lemon juice, garlic clove, salt, cumin and pepper to a food processor and blend on high until smooth and creamy.

5. Transfer to a serving bowl and garnish with the toasted sunflower seeds and chopped coriander.

If your cauliflower hummus is a bit thick, just add more water (a teaspoon at a time) until you get the desired level of creaminess.

I large head of cauliflower
4 tbsp olive oil
A handful of sunflower seeds
4 tbsp tahini paste (light or dark)
2 tbsp water, or more
    for desired consistency
Juice of I lemon
I garlic clove
½ tsp salt
¼ tsp ground cumin
Black pepper, to taste
A handful of chopped
    fresh coriander, to serve

SIDES + DRESSINGS

Broccamoley

This delicious mash-up of broccoli and guacamole is packed with potassium, liver-supporting nutrients, healthy fats and B vitamins – the perfect accompaniment to baked fish, roast chicken legs, pan-fried steak or simply served with sauerkraut.

I head of broccoli
I ripe avocado, peeled
   and stoned
3 tbsp nutritional yeast,
   plus extra for serving
I garlic clove
½ tsp salt
2 tbsp natural or
   coconut yoghurt

1. Cut the broccoli into florets.

2. Steam the broccoli for 6 minutes until tender but still green. Run under cold water to stop the cooking process.

3. Add the broccoli with all the other ingredients to a blender and roughly combine, leaving some texture.

4. Plate up and add an additional sprinkling of nutritional yeast.

SIDES + DRESSINGS

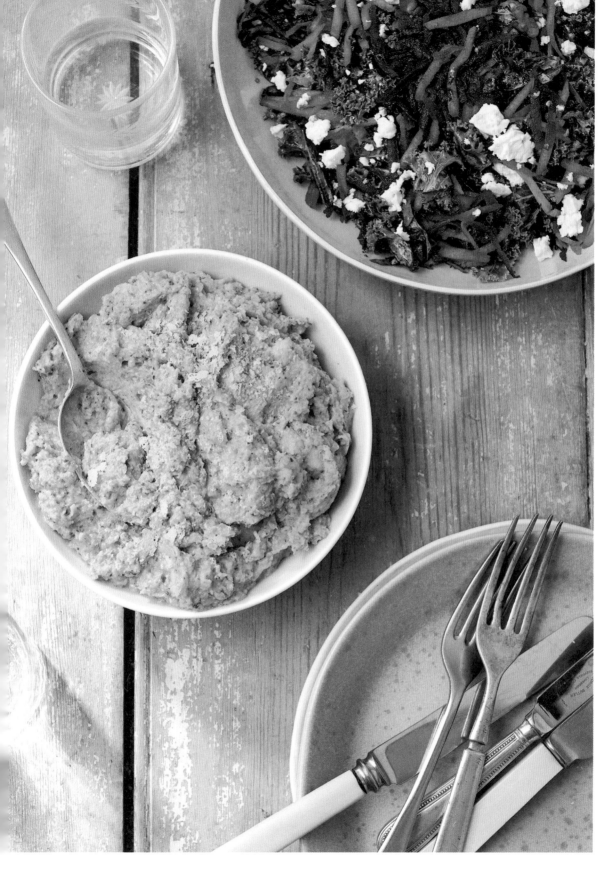

Smoked salmon & prawn mousse in minutes

This fail-safe mousse is packed with protein, anti-inflammatory fats and the hormone hero, magnesium. It works as a protein-packed, super low-carb breakfast or a light lunch.

30g ghee or butter
8 large eggs
100ml cream, milk
    or unsweetened nut milk
100g smoked salmon
Small bunch of fresh chives,
    chopped
2 spring onions
150g cooked peeled prawns
Salt and black pepper, to taste
1 lemon, cut into 4 wedges,
    to serve

1. Melt the ghee or butter in a frying pan, then crack in the eggs and cook to scramble them. Take off the heat to cool slightly.

2. Add the slightly cooled scrambled eggs, cream or milk, salt and pepper to a blender and combine until smooth and creamy.

3. Add three-quarters of the smoked salmon to the blender and pulse until the mixture is speckled with salmon pieces. Mix in the chopped chives, reserving some to garnish.

4. Chop the spring onions into thin slivers and then toss evenly into four ramekins.

5. Spoon the egg and salmon mix into the ramekins and allow to set in the fridge for 3–4 hours.

6. Layer the mousse with cooked prawns, slivers of the remaining salmon and serve each with a lemon wedge, with the reserved chives sprinkled over.

This mousse works well without the prawns, too!

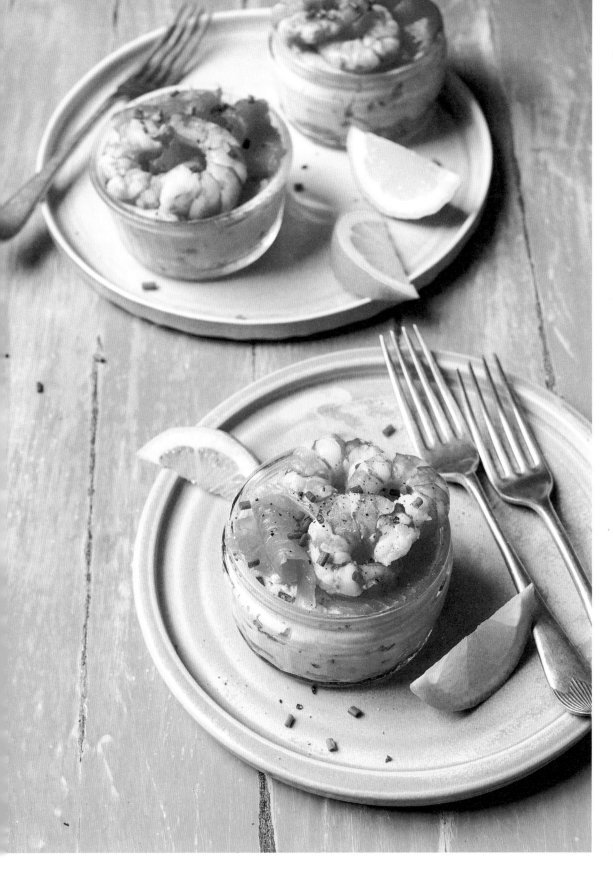

Chicken soup for the soul

Chicken bone broth makes the most wonderful base for many a dish. Packed with bone-strengthening, muscle-building and skin-loving ingredients, bone broth is a girl's best friend!

I roasted chicken carcass
(ideally a free-range organic)
2–3 chicken feet (if your
butcher has them!)
I large onion, unpeeled
and roughly chopped.
2 heads of garlic, unpeeled
4 celery stalks, unpeeled
and chopped into quarters
4 medium carrots, chopped
into quarters
2 tbsp garlic powder
I tbsp ground turmeric
2 dried bay leaves
1½ tbsp apple cider vinegar
2½ tsp Himalayan rock salt
Black pepper, to taste

1. Add all of the ingredients to a slow cooker or a large pan on the hob. Add enough water to cover the chicken carcass and cook at a low setting for 12 hours. Check occasionally, and if your water levels become low, top up with extra water.

2. Allow the broth to cool. Keep some broth with veggies in to serve as soup, but strain the remainder, pour into ice-cube trays and freeze for up to 6 months.

See Chilled & creamy avo soup (page 178) for a delicious meal in minutes made using chicken broth.

Bread + Buns

The best buns

These buns are bursting with fibre and vitamin E. They are low in carbs, ideal for stabilising blood sugar levels and keeping hunger at bay.

30g chia seeds, ground
30g golden linseeds, ground
30g sesame seeds, ground,
    plus extra seeds to top
150g coconut flour
100g almond flour
150g psyllium husk
4 tsp baking powder
1½ tsp salt
10ml apple cider vinegar
6 eggs
60g coconut oil
750ml water

1. Preheat the oven to 170°C fan.

2. Add the ground seeds to a mixing bowl and rub together until the mixture resembles an evenly coloured sand, then stirring in the psyllium husk, baking powder and salt.

3. Mix all of the wet ingredients together before combining this with the dry mix, stirring with a spoon to form a dough. It will look very odd when you initially add all of the liquid to the dry, but the psyllium husk will very quickly absorb the moisture and turn it into a rather interesting Play-Doh consistency!

4. Create apple-sized balls of dough by rolling the mix in your hands (rubbing your hands in melted coconut oil helps to create smoother rolls!).

5. Place the dough balls onto a lined baking sheet and sprinkle with the extra sesame seeds. Bake for 45 minutes.

Allow to cool before slicing and freezing, or store in the fridge for 5 days.

BREAD + BUNS

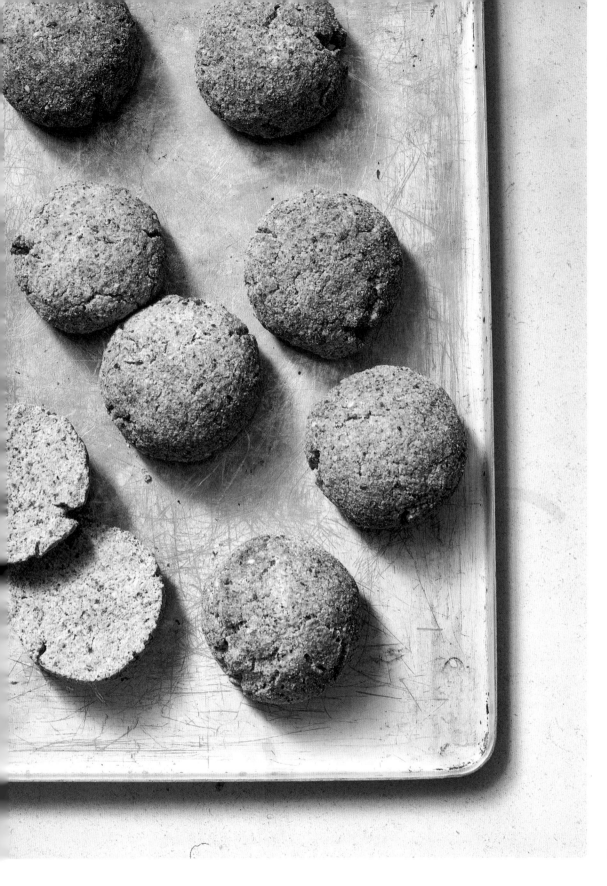

Back atcha focaccia!

This low-carb version of an Italian classic is the bread that keeps on giving! Full of healthy fats and the aromatic flavour of rosemary, you'll be high-fiving yourself when this beauty comes out of the oven. With thanks to Hunter & Gather for this fabulous recipe.

2 tbsp cream cheese
350g grated mozzarella cheese
150g ground almonds
1 tbsp baking powder
1 large egg
Hunter & Gather extra virgin
    olive oil, for drizzling
1 tsp coarse sea salt
1 sprig of fresh rosemary, leaves
    roughly chopped

1. Preheat the oven to 175°C fan and select a 20cm square baking dish.

2. Add the cream cheese and mozzarella to a microwave-safe bowl and heat in 30-second increments until melted, stirring between each heating.

3. Once melted, allow to cool slightly before adding the ground almonds, baking powder and egg – use your hands to mix together until a cohesive dough is formed.

4. Press the dough into an even layer in the dish, making sure to cover it with the traditional focaccia-style dimples, using your fingertips.

5. Drizzle the dough with olive oil and sprinkle generously with sea salt and fresh rosemary.

6. Bake for 20–25 minutes until golden brown, then allow to cool slightly before slicing and enjoying.

BREAD + BUNS

Fibre-rich flatbreads

These are the *ultimate* in fibre-packed goodness. Psyllium husk is a liver-loving, gut-happy ingredient that will help you feel fuller for longer and keep your digestive health in tip-top shape.

30g butter or coconut oil, melted
5 tbsp coconut flour
3 tbsp psyllium husk
2 tbsp ground almonds
1 egg
1 tsp baking powder
1 tsp xanthan gum
½ tsp salt

1. Add the butter or coconut oil to a frying pan and gently melt. Transfer most of this melted butter or oil to a mixing bowl (leaving a little in the pan).

2. Add all other ingredients to the mixing bowl and combine to form a dough.

3. Split the mixture into 3–4 equal amounts. Roll each into a ball and flatten in the palm of your hand. Transfer the flattened dough to the hot, oiled pan.

4. Fry on each side for 3–4 minutes until golden brown.

Serve with a dollop of coconut yoghurt, a sprinkle of beetroot salt, smoked salmon and mashed avocado. Delicious!

Glazed low-carb teacakes

A low-carb version of a teacake, toasted with a little goat's butter or nut butter, delicious!

The Best buns mix (see page 170)

PLUS
3 tsp ground cinnamon
1½ tsp ground ginger
Juice and zest of 1 unwaxed orange
A handful of chopped pecans
A handful of golden sultanas
3–4 tbsp low-sugar apricot fruit spread
Zest of 1 unwaxed lemon

1. Preheat the oven to 170°C fan.

2. Instead of using water as per the Best buns recipe, you can use nut milk for additional richness (you don't have to, they still work well with water). Make the buns as per the Best buns recipe, only this time add the spices, orange zest, chopped nuts and sultanas.

3. Bake for 45 minutes as per the Best buns recipe.

4. Remove the teacakes from the oven and leave to cool.

5. Meanwhile, make the glaze. In a saucepan, gently warm the apricot spread with 2 tablespoons of water. Using a pastry brush, glaze the teacakes and sprinkle with the lemon zest. Refrigerate for up to 5 days or freeze for up to 3 months.

Low-carb loaf

This seed-flour bread is full of protein and fibre, the ideal combo for keeping you feeling full, and it won't raise your blood sugars like wheat bread will!

150g golden linseeds
150g sunflower seeds
I heaped tsp gluten-free
     baking powder
I tsp salt
5 eggs, beaten
I good capful of apple
     cider vinegar
40g coconut oil, ghee
     or butter, melted

1.   Preheat the oven to 170°C fan. Line a 450g loaf tin with parchment paper (or the loaf tin liner inserts you can buy are super handy!)

2.   Grind up the golden linseeds in a blender or food processor, then tip into a large mixing bowl. Do the same with the sunflower seeds.

3.   Add the baking powder and salt to the mixing bowl and combine well using your hands, rubbing the ground seeds together.

4.   Add the beaten eggs, apple cider vinegar and melted oil or butter and mix. The batter will become quite thick and sticky.

5.   Transfer the mix into the lined tin and bake for 30–35 minutes.

6.   Remove and allow to cool.

Serve toasted with a slather of goat's butter … delicious! Slice up and freeze individual pieces for handy low-carb bread when you need a quick scrambled eggs or mashed avo on toast!

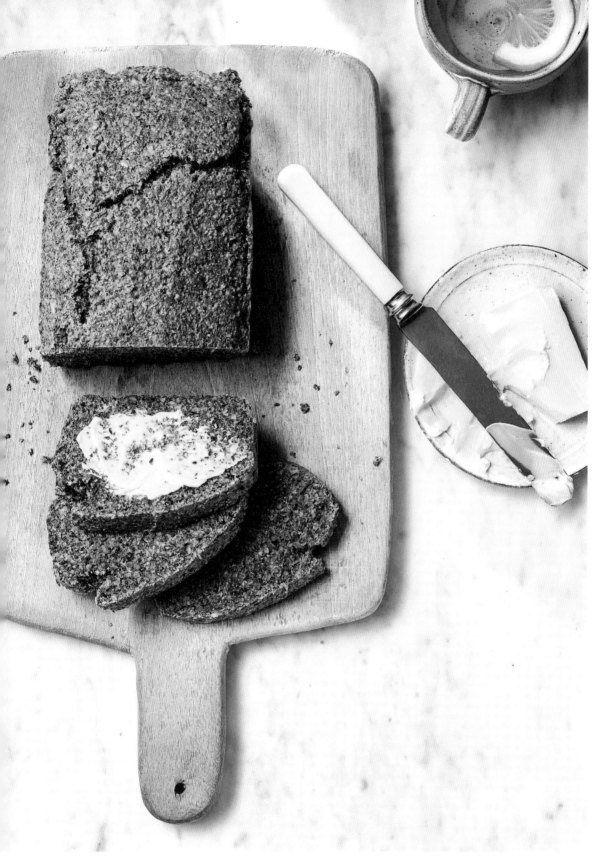

Loaded Italian loaf

This low-carb loaf is loaded with flavour and goodness. Toasted and slathered in butter or eaten cold with some salad leaves and sauerkraut, it is the perfect fridge staple for a busy day!

220g ground almonds
2 heaped tsp baking powder
½ tsp salt
Black pepper (generous grind)
1 tsp dried mixed herbs
4 eggs, beaten
60g butter or ghee, melted
100g feta cheese, crumbled
    into large pieces
100g red pepper, deseeded
    and chopped
100g spring onions, chopped

1. Preheat the oven to 175°C fan. Line a 450g loaf tin with parchment paper (or the loaf tin liner inserts you can buy are super handy!)

2. Mix the dry ingredients together in a bowl.

3. Add the eggs and melted butter and stir to combine.

4. Add the cheese, red pepper and spring onions, stir until just combined and place into the tin without pressing down. It will look as if there isn't enough batter to cover the veg and cheese, but don't worry, everything will fuse together as it cooks.

5. Bake for 45 minutes, until golden on top and springy to touch. Leave to cool in the tin for a little while, then turn out on a wire rack and cool.

Once you've mastered the basic recipe you can vary the flavours to suit what's in season, what you have available and whatever is to your taste. Try swapping feta for goat's cheese or blue cheese, switch spring onion for rocket or spinach.

Main Meals

Chilled & creamy avo soup

Crème de la crème tomato soup

This is the ultimate 'meal-in-minutes' and go-to for a mega-dose of nutrients! Packed with calcium, magnesium, potassium and a whole spectrum of vitamins, this super soup is both delicious and nutritious. Homemade bone broth with some leftover veggies works really well for this recipe. Alternatively, use a store-bought bone broth with veggies, such as the Ossa range.

When you're in a hurry and need a nutritious soup that takes no time (at all!) to make, this soup hits the mark every time. Mixing up a few store-cupboard essentials means this meal is ready in minutes.

400ml bone broth (homemade, see page 159, or from your store cupboard/fridge)
250ml jar of passata or a jar of pasta sauce (see page 83)
2 Best buns (see page 170)

TOPPER IDEAS
Seeds, chopped herbs, drizzle of olive oil, balsamic vinegar, kefir, sauerkraut, nutritional yeast, crack of black pepper, garlic salt …

250ml chicken or beef bone broth (use homemade, see page 159, or use store-bought)
1 ripe avocado, peeled and stoned
1 Best bun (page 170, optional)
A drizzle of olive oil
A drizzle of balsamic vinegar

TO SERVE
Chopped fresh herbs/dehydrated kale chips/ nutritional yeast
A good pinch of beetroot salt

1. Warm the bone broth and passata or pasta sauce together in a large pan.

2. Add the warmed mix to a blender and add one of the Best buns, chopped up. Combine until smooth, thick and creamy.

3. Pour into two bowls and top with seeds, herbs, oil, balsamic vinegar, a drizzle of kefir, a spoonful of sauerkraut – any toppers to upgrade your soup! Serve with the remaining Best bun.

1. Add the bone broth to a blender (cold from the fridge or tepid from the cupboard, do not heat).

2. Add the avocado and blend with the bone broth until smooth and creamy. If your bone broth has veggies in, the soup will be thicker; if it's a clear broth, it won't thicken as much. You can add half a Best bun to the mix to thicken the soup further, using the other half to dunk into the soup.

3. Pour into a bowl and drizzle with olive oil and balsamic vinegar, then sprinkle with herbs, dehydrated kale or nutritional yeast and some beetroot salt and serve with the remaining half, if you like.

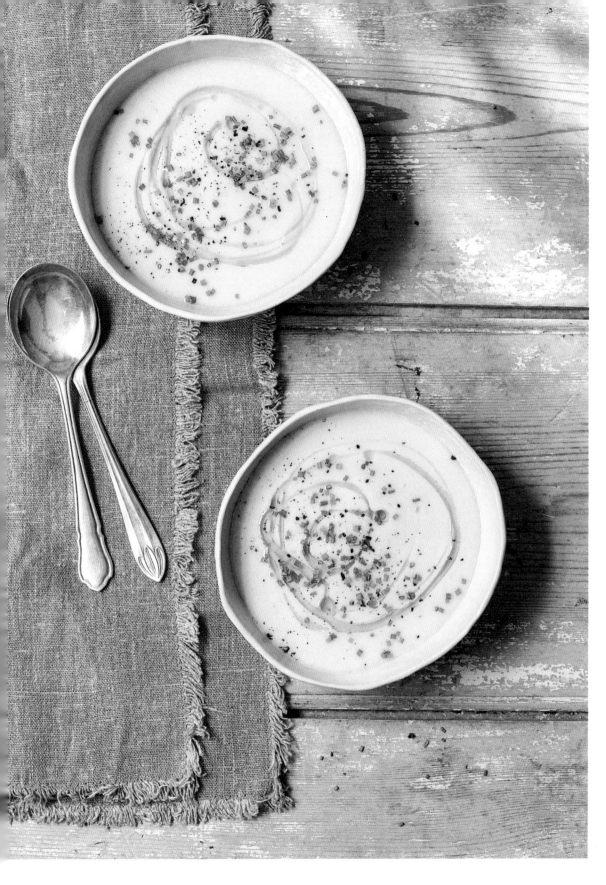

Roquefort, rocket & pink grapefruit salad

As colourful in nutrients as it is in appearance, this easy-to-construct salad is a powerhouse of goodness!

90g rocket
100g Roquefort (ideally raw), cut into chunks
1 ripe avocado, peeled, stoned and sliced
2 pink grapefruits, segmented
A drizzle of Black tahini & miso dressing (see page 150)
A handful of chopped fresh coriander
A handful of pecans, chopped
A handful of sunflower seeds

1. Lay the rocket leaves onto two plates, adding chunks of Roquefort, slices of avocado and pink grapefruit segments and drizzle over the Black tahini & miso dressing.

2. Sprinkle over the chopped coriander, pecans and sunflower seeds.

Add in a slice of toasted Low-carb loaf (page 174) for an extra hit of fibre and to keep you feeling fuller for longer.

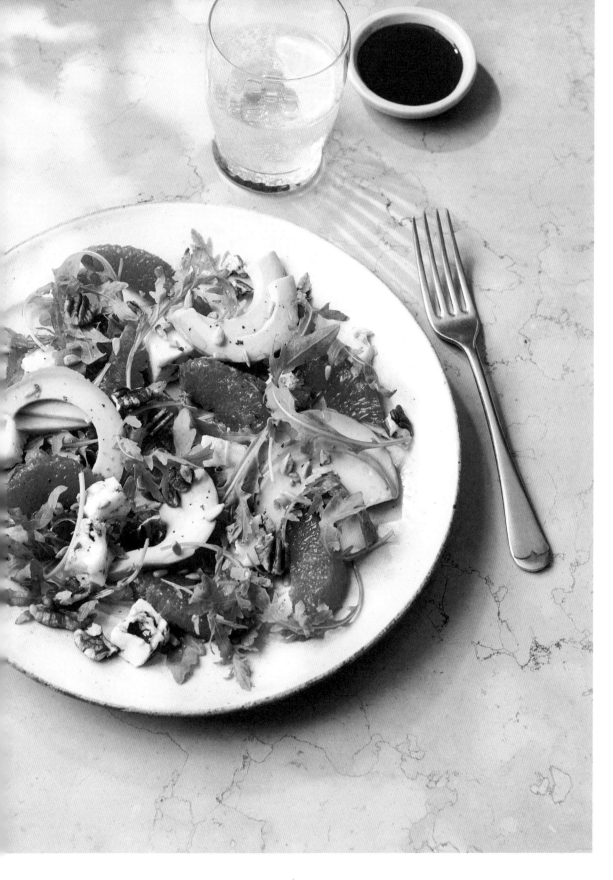

Five-minute mushroom stroganoff

Mushrooms have wonderful medicinal properties, and each variety offers a host of benefits. From the humble button to the masterful Lion's Mane, add any mushrooms you have to hand to this recipe.

500g mushrooms
(chestnut, button,
mixed wild mushrooms)
Coconut oil, for frying
1 generous tbsp miso paste
300ml coconut yoghurt
2 tbsp coconut aminos
300g Turmeric & coconut
cauli-rice (see page 144)
or a packet of store-bought
cauliflower rice, to serve
A handful of chopped
fresh coriander, to garnish

1. Sauté the mushrooms in a pan with the coconut oil and miso until golden and soft. Add the yoghurt and coconut aminos and warm through.

2. Warm the Turmeric & coconut cauli-rice for 5–6 minutes in the oven (or follow the instructions on the packet if using store-bought) before serving with the mushroom stroganoff, sprinkled with the chopped coriander.

For additional protein, add sliced chicken to the sautéed mushrooms or serve with a beef steak and salad leaves.

Baked avocados with a cheesy herb crust

Healthy doesn't get much more satisfying than this! A firm favourite on the fast-food front, packed with flavour and satisfyingly delicious. Once bitten, forever smitten!

1. Preheat the oven to 180°C fan.

2. Place the four avocado halves onto a baking dish. Using a teaspoon, make the hole from the stone in the avocado a little larger by scooping out just a little flesh. Sprinkle a little salt onto the avocado flesh.

3. Crack the eggs, separating the whites and yolks, adding the yolks to the hole in the avocado halves. Pop the whites in the fridge or freezer for another recipe.

4. Add the cubed cheese, roughly chopped bread and the herbs to a blender and pulse for 60 seconds until finely combined cheesy breadcrumbs form.

5. Carefully pile the breadcrumb mix in a mound on top of the eggs, trying not to break the yolks. Bake in the oven for 15 minutes.

Eat hot or cold, an ideal picnic food or packed lunch that will keep you feeling full and satisfied!

2 ripe avocados, peeled,
   cut in half and stoned
A pinch of salt
4 eggs
40g hard cheese of choice
   (goat's Cheddar works well),
   cut into rough cubes
1 Best bun (see page 170) or
   2 slices of Low-carb loaf (see
   page 174), roughly chopped
1 tbsp mixed dried herbs

MAIN MEALS

Creamy curried cauli steaks

Cauliflower is your liver's best friend when it comes to detoxification, supporting the removal of used hormones and waste products. A well-functioning liver is better for blood sugars and hormonal balance.

I large head of cauliflower
I heaped tsp miso paste
I tsp salt
2 garlic cloves, diced
400ml tin of coconut milk
Coconut oil, for frying
2 tsp curry powder

TO SERVE
A handful of chopped fresh
   coriander
A handful of slivered almonds
A handful of pomegranate seeds
A pinch of beetroot salt

1. Preheat the oven to 180°C fan.

2. Prepare the cauliflower by removing the base and leaves. Set these to one side while you slice the cauliflower into 2cm thick steaks. Place the cauliflower steaks in an ovenproof dish.

3. Return to the cauliflower base, remove the central stalk, discarding the leaves. Slice the central stalk, which slightly resembles celery, into thin pieces.

4. In a pan, heat the coconut oil and add the curry powder, miso paste, salt, thinly sliced cauliflower stalks and diced garlic and allow to cook for 3–4 minutes. Add the coconut milk and stir to combine.

5. Pour the curry-coconut mix on top of the cauliflower steaks, spooning over to ensure maximum coverage. Bake for 40–45 minutes until tender.

6. Remove from the oven, sprinkle with chopped coriander, almond slivers, pomegranate seeds and beetroot salt.

Serve with salad leaves, Lemon olive oil mayonnaise (see page 151) or Roasted red pepper pesto (see page 152) and sauerkraut.

MAIN MEALS

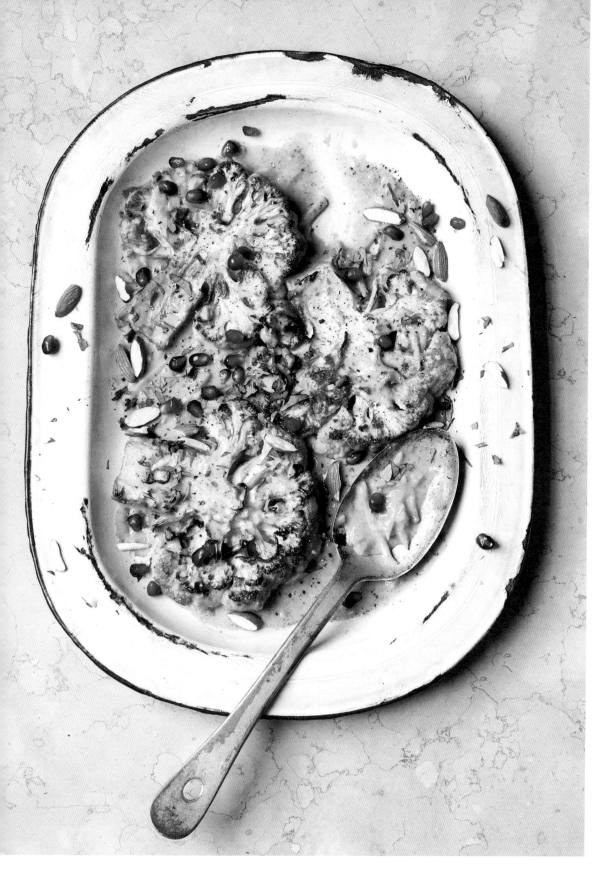

Tickled pink pickled egg salad

This dish is as pretty as a picture and packed with nutrients to support gut health and energy levels. With a few fridge essentials and a little advance preparation, making the eggs 2–3 days ahead, it takes just a few minutes to put together.

3–4 hard-boiled eggs, cooled and shelled
Beet kvass (homemade, see page 110 or store-bought)
Raspberry blush vinaigrette (see page 148) or 1 tbsp mayonnaise
100g salad leaves of choice
A handful of roughly chopped pecans
A handful of chopped fresh chives
A handful of pomegranate seeds

1. First prep the eggs. Place the eggs into a clean glass jar and fill with Beet kvass until the eggs are covered. Place in the fridge for 2–3 days. To firm up the eggs before pickling, they can be placed in a freezer bag with salt overnight to draw out the water and increase firmness. This step isn't essential, it just results in firmer eggs!

2. Once the eggs have been sat in the Beet kvass for a few days, remove and slice them in half and place to one side. Make the Raspberry blush vinaigrette (unless you have it already in the fridge!), or if you're in a hurry, use a spoonful of mayo as an alternative.

3. Add salad leaves to your plate, placing the sliced pink egg halves on top of the leaves before spooning on as much vinaigrette as you like and sprinkling with chopped pecans, chives and pomegranate seeds.

To bump up this salad, add slices of ripe avocado sprinkled with salt.

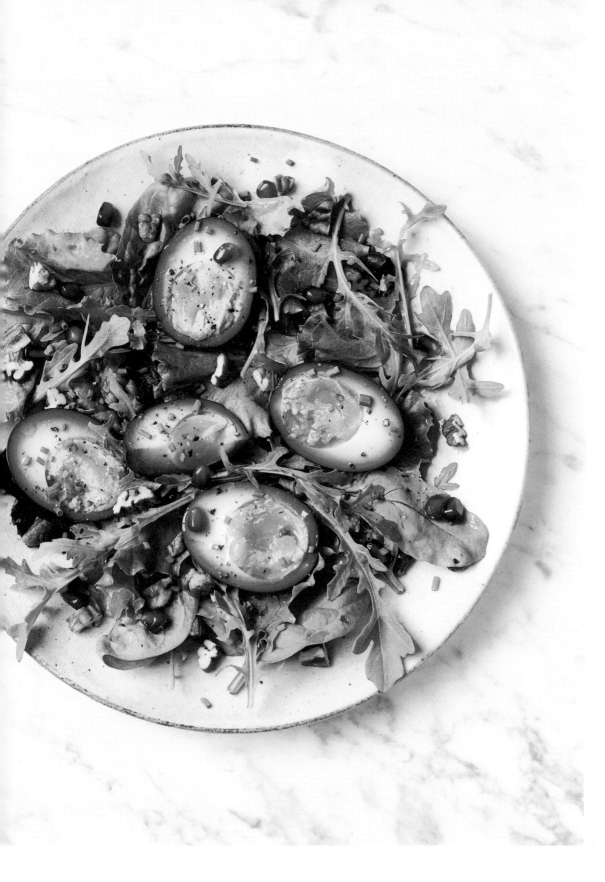

Spiced cauli-lamb meatballs in miso pepper passata

These flavoursome meatballs are packed with the goodness of cauliflower, minced lamb and spices, and served submerged in a rich red pepper and miso tomato sauce, finished with tangy feta.

Olive oil or butter, for frying
1 tsp miso paste
2 tsp smoked paprika
2 garlic cloves
200g cauliflower rice
    (homemade, see page 143,
    or store-bought)
1 egg
400g lamb mince
1 tsp onion granules
2 tsp dried mixed herbs
Salt and black pepper, to taste

FOR THE SAUCE
Ghee or butter, for frying
1 onion, diced
1 red pepper, deseeded
    and chopped
1 tsp miso paste
2 garlic cloves, finely chopped
700ml of passata
2 cubes of Bone broth (see
    page 159, optional)
1 tsp dried mixed herbs

TO SERVE
Fresh coriander
Crumbled feta cheese
Sauerkraut

1. To make the meatballs, add a little olive oil or butter to a pan and heat. Next add the miso paste, paprika, garlic, 1 teaspoon of salt and the cauliflower rice and sauté for 3–4 minutes.

2. In a mixing bowl, add the egg, lamb mince, onion granules, mixed herbs and black pepper. Transfer the cauliflower mix to the lamb and combine, shaping the mix into 15 plum-sized balls. Refrigerate for 15–20 minutes while you prepare the sauce.

3. Add a little ghee or butter to a heavy-based pan (that has a lid) and gently fry the onion, red pepper, miso and garlic. Add the passata, cubes of Bone broth, if using, dried herbs and 200ml of water. Season with salt and pepper and simmer for 10 minutes.

4. Place the chilled meatballs into the pan of tomato sauce, cover with a lid and cook on a medium heat for 20 minutes.

5. Serve in pasta bowls sprinkled with coriander and feta cheese, alongside sauerkraut.

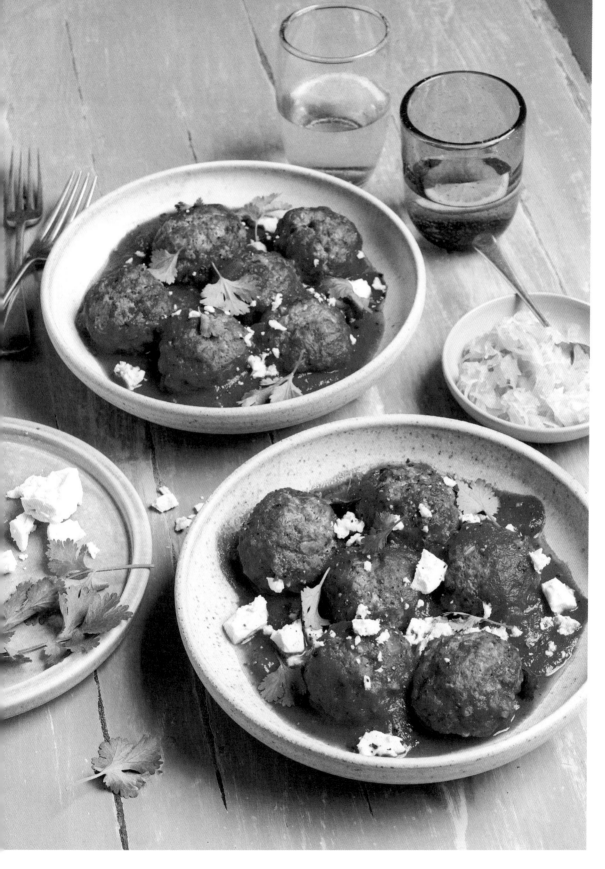

Super green cauli-rice risotto

Risotto … with a difference. This fibre-packed, low-carb version of a classic is speedy, delicious and healthy, full of potassium and magnesium and liver-loving goodness.

Coconut oil, for frying
1 white onion, diced
1 garlic clove, minced
1 leek, sliced and washed
2 small courgettes, chopped
400g cauli-rice (plain, raw
    Cauli-rice, page 143,
    or store-bought)
150ml veggie stock or
    bone broth or 4 ice cubes
    of frozen bone broth
½ bag of spinach
½ bag of kale, chopped
    with stalks removed
30g nutritional yeast,
    plus extra to serve
A drizzle of olive oil
A handful of sunflower
    seeds and pumpkin seeds
Chopped fresh herbs of choice
A good pinch of beetroot salt
    or sea salt

1. Add a little coconut oil into a large pan and sauté the onions, garlic, leek and courgettes until soft and brown. Add in the cauli-rice and cook with the veggie mix for a few minutes before adding the stock.

2. Add the spinach and chopped kale, allowing it to wilt into the cauli-rice mix.

3. Take half of the veggie-cauli mix and add to a blender, then combine until smooth.

4. Reintroduce the smooth mix back to the remaining half of the veggie-cauli mix and stir in the nutritional yeast before plating up.

5. Drizzle with olive oil, toss on the seeds and chopped herbs, beetroot salt and an extra sprinkle of nutritional yeast.

Add a dollop of Roasted red pepper pesto for an extra kick (see page 152).

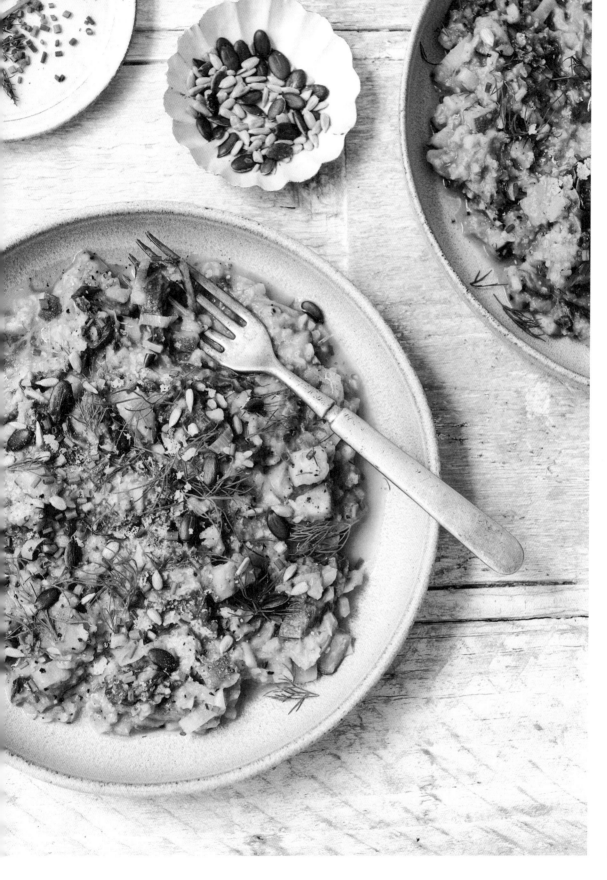

Smokey chicken drumsticks with roasted red pepper pesto

This powerhouse of a dish is packed with protein, a fermented dressing bursting with goodness, skin-saviour vitamin E, liver-loving garlic and potassium-rich basil. Replace the chicken with organic tofu for a vegan alternative.

1 heaped tbsp ghee
   or coconut oil
2 tsp smoked paprika
1 tsp salt
2 tsp onion powder
4 red onions
6–8 chicken drumsticks
2 red peppers, deseeded
   and roughly chopped

ROASTED RED PEPPER PESTO
60ml olive oil
15ml apple cider vinegar
1 tsp salt
1 garlic clove
1 tsp miso paste
30g sunflower seeds
A handful of fresh basil

TO SERVE
A handful of salad leaves
A forkful of sauerkraut

1. Preheat the oven to 180°C fan.

2. Melt the ghee or coconut oil in a pan, add the smoked paprika, salt and onion powder and gently sauté for 1–3 minutes. Turn off the heat.

3. Slice the red onions in half, keeping the skins on, then place cut side down in a large ovenproof dish.

4. Add the chicken to a mixing bowl, pat dry and add to the peppers. Pour in the paprika and oil mix then, using your hands, coat the chicken and peppers in the paprika, onion and oil mix before adding them to the ovenproof dish with the onions. Roast for 40–45 minutes until the skin is golden and crispy.

5. Remove from the oven and add half of the roasted peppers, some of the juices from the baking tray and all of the pesto ingredients, except the basil, to a blender and combine until smooth and creamy. Add the basil and pulse.

6. Squeeze the red onions out of their skins onto plates along with the remaining peppers, adding a handful of salad leaves, a forkful of sauerkraut and the chicken legs, dolloping on the pesto. Devour!

This recipe also works well with chicken thighs, however, cooking times may need to be adjusted.

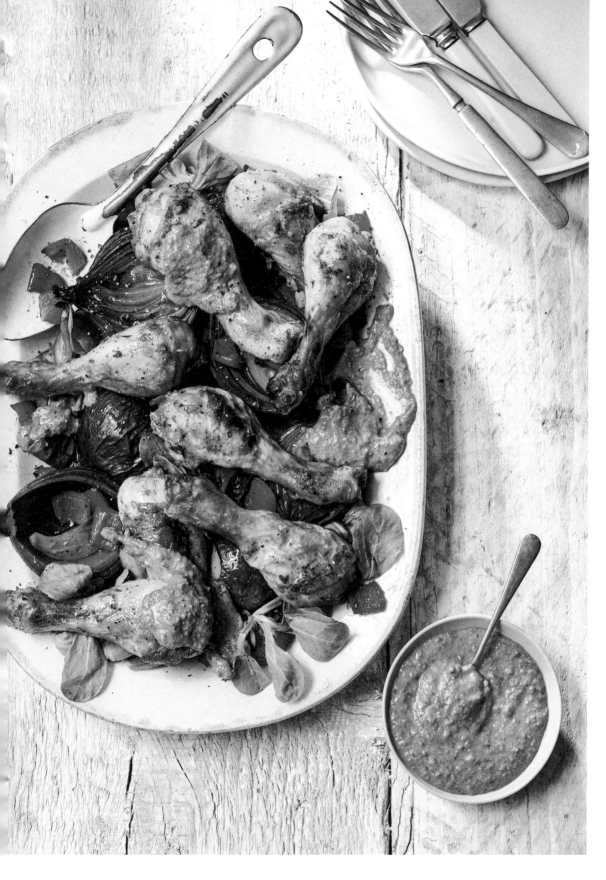

Kale, feta, walnut & pomegranate salad

Crumbly fresh feta works a treat with the jewels of sweet pomegranate and the deep tahini salad dressing. The pumpkin seeds are a rich source of zinc, for glowing skin and a healthy immune system.

2 carrots
2 beetroots
I bag of kale, stalks removed
½ quantity of Black
    tahini & miso dressing
    (page 150)
I small red onion, diced
A handful of chopped walnuts
I ripe avocado, peeled,
    stoned and sliced
100g feta cheese, cut into cubes
A handful of pomegranate seeds
A handful of pumpkin seeds

1. Start by grating the carrots and beetroot (keeping the skin on for extra fibre) into a bowl and placing to one side.

2. Chop the kale and cut into bite-size pieces. Place in a large mixing bowl.

3. Pour in the Black tahini & miso dressing and rub it into the kale, giving it a good massage for 5–6 minutes.

4. Next add the grated veggies, diced red onion and chopped walnuts to the mix and toss around in the oily dressing.

5. Place the kale-carrot-beet mix into a pasta-style bowl. Layer on the sliced avocado, cubed feta cheese and finish with the pomegranate seeds and pumpkin seeds.

MAIN MEALS

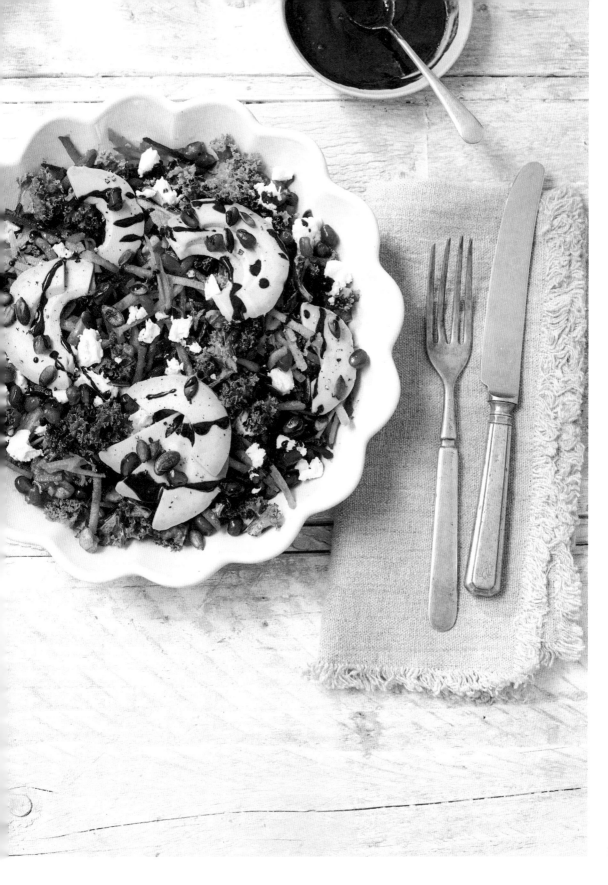

No time to cook aubergine bake

Well-intentioned habits can start to slip when we are just too tired or busy to cook. This simple five-minute meal takes very little preparation and is packed with phytonutrients and fibre, perfect for replenishing energy levels.

2 large, firm aubergines
8 tbsp natural or
    coconut yoghurt
2 tsp miso paste
2 tbsp coconut aminos
A few cracks of black pepper
A pinch of beetroot salt
    or sea salt

TO SERVE
Finely sliced spring onions,
    to serve
A handful of pomegranate
    seeds, to serve

1. Preheat the oven to 180°C fan.

2. Start by slicing the aubergines in half, lengthways, to create aubergine boats.

3. Score the flesh in a crisscross manner, being careful not to cut too deep, and keep the skin of the aubergine intact at the base.

4. In a small bowl, combine the yoghurt, miso, coconut aminos, black pepper and salt.

5. Place the aubergine in an ovenproof dish. Spoon half of the yoghurt-miso dressing onto the scored side of the aubergine boats and bake facing upwards for 40–60 minutes, depending on the size of the aubergines, until soft and tender.

6. Once baked, place the aubergine boats on to your plates and drizzle over the remaining yoghurt-miso dressing mix, adding the finely chopped spring onions and pomegranate seeds.

Serve with salad leaves and kimchi/sauerkraut.

Bean so busy ... pasta bake

No fuss, low carb and high in protein, this rich tomato and bean pasta bake is a go-to when the fridge is looking a little bare and you have just been too busy to think about dinner!

1. Preheat the oven to 180°C fan.

2. Add the dried pasta to an ovenproof dish.

3. Combine the jar of pasta sauce with the bone broth or veggie stock in a jug and pour over the pasta, making sure the pasta is submerged. Cover with the grated cheese, if using.

4. Bake for 25 minutes until bubbling and the cheese is golden brown.

Serve with salad leaves and a forkful of sauerkraut.

150g bean pasta (Edamame & Mung Bean Fettuccine by Explore Cuisine works brilliantly, widely available)

400g jar of no-added-sugar pasta sauce (Seggiano sauces are delicious)

400ml bone broth or veggie stock

50g grated Cheddar (optional)

MAIN MEALS

Beetroot-salted steak, macadamia nuts & raspberry blush vinaigrette

This simple steak is elevated to tangy heights with the addition of the Raspberry blush vinaigrette.

2 beef steaks of choice
Ghee, butter or olive oil,
    for frying
100g of mixed leaves
1 red onion, thinly sliced
A handful of salted
    macadamia nuts
Raspberry blush vinaigrette
    (see page 148)
A good pinch of beetroot salt

1. Start by taking the steaks out of the fridge 30 minutes prior to cooking.

2. Next, heat a pan and add some ghee, butter or olive oil. Get the pan nice and hot before adding the steak and cooking it on one side for 2–3 minutes (depending on how you like it cooked). Don't touch it while it cooks.

3. Meanwhile, place the prepared leaves onto plates and toss over the sliced red onion.

4. Turn the steak and cook on the other side for 2–3 minutes before removing from the heat and leaving to rest for 15–20 minutes.

5. Slice the steaks on a 45-degree angle and place on the plates. Sprinkle over the macadamia nuts, generously drizzle over the vinaigrette and finish with a good pinch of beetroot salt.

Serve with sauerkraut, avocado slices or Lemon olive oil mayonnaise (see page 151).

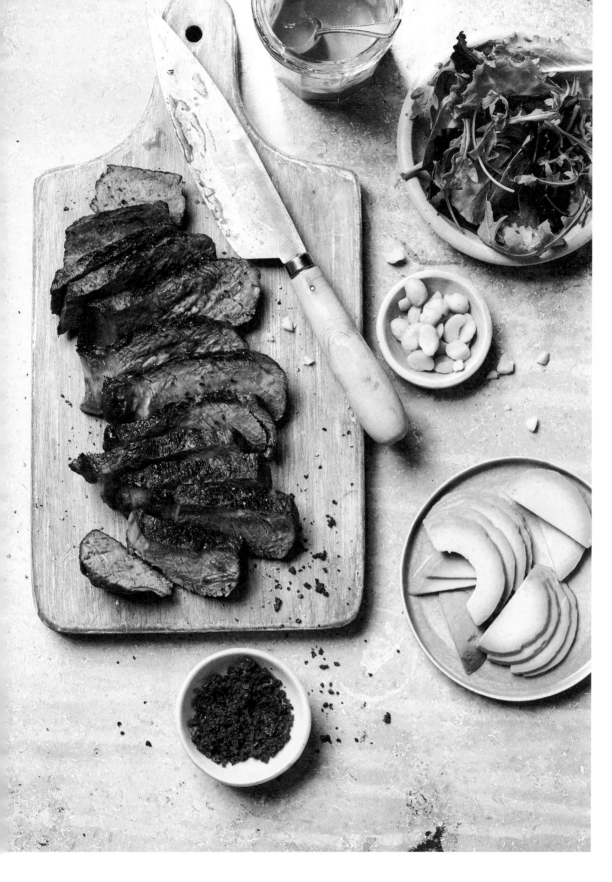

Double beetroot salad with crumbled feta & leafy greens

Beetroot is packed with naturally occurring nitrates, which boost the skin-benefiting compound, nitric oxide. This recipe incorporates the beneficial bacteria from fermented Beet kvass within the vinaigrette and the rich sweetness of roasted beetroot.

6–8 raw beetroots (or double up for making extras for other recipes)
Coconut oil or ghee, for roasting
1 head of broccoli
A handful of pumpkin seeds
A few sunflower seeds
Raspberry blush vinaigrette (see page 148)
Some salad leaves of choice
60g feta cheese, crumbled
A pinch of beetroot salt or sea salt

1. Preheat the oven to 180°C fan.

2. Cut each beetroot into chunks of 6–8 pieces. Place them in an ovenproof dish and cover with coconut oil or ghee and roast for 40–45 minutes until soft.

3. While the beetroots are roasting, cut the broccoli into florets and steam (ideally) or boil until they are tender. Remove from the steamer or pan, drain and run under cold water to stop further cooking.

4. In a large bowl, toss together the roast beetroot, broccoli, pumpkin seeds and sunflower seeds and combine with as much Raspberry blush vinaigrette as you like. Plate up the leaves and beetroot salad, adding the crumbled feta and a sprinkle of beetroot salt.

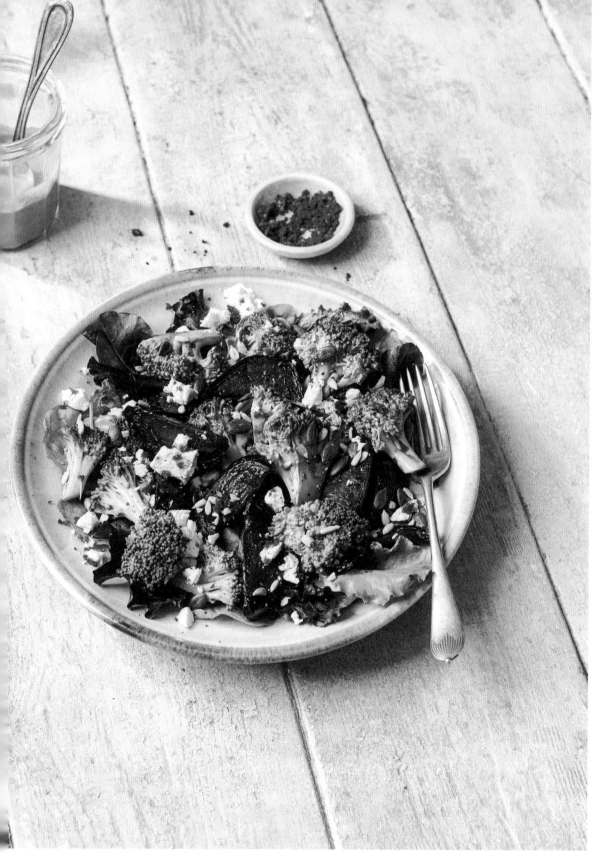

Egg-fried prawn cauli-rice

This low-carb, protein- and fibre-packed meal takes minutes to make and is, surprisingly, just like the 'real deal'!

Ghee or coconut oil, for frying
1 tsp miso paste
2 spring onions, finely chopped
2 carrots, finely chopped
1 tsp pre-chopped ginger
   or grated fresh ginger
120g frozen edamame beans
200g cooked and peeled prawns
400g cauliflower rice (see page
   143 or store-bought)
3 eggs
2 tbsp coconut aminos,
   plus extra to serve
1 tsp salt or garlic salt
Fresh coriander
1 tbsp sesame seeds

1. Melt a dollop of ghee or coconut oil in a wok or frying pan and add the miso paste.

2. Add the spring onions, keeping a little back for serving, and carrots to the pan along with the ginger and sauté for 3–4 minutes.

3. Add the edamame beans and continue to cook for a further 2–3 minutes before adding the prawns and cauliflower rice and cook for a further 2–3 minutes.

4. In the meantime, beat the eggs together. Make a small well in the centre of the prawn-cauli mix and pour in the eggs. Let the eggs set before stirring in.

5. Add in the coconut aminos and salt and mix before plating up. Sprinkle with the reserved spring onion, fresh coriander, sesame seeds and a drizzle of coconut aminos.

Serve with a side of kimchi.

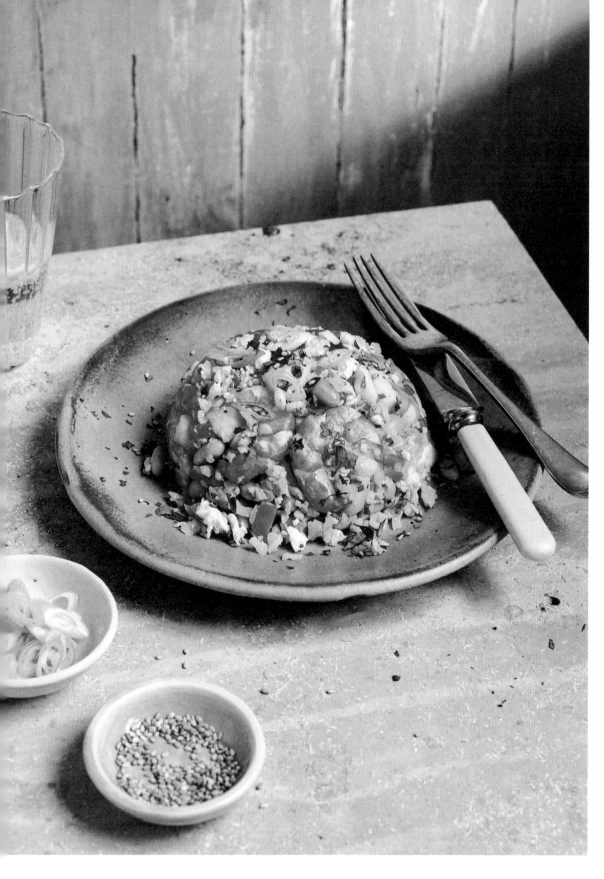

Minced beef ... three ways

Beef is one of the most nutrient-rich foods on the planet, packed with protein, B vitamins, selenium (needed for healthy thyroid function), zinc, copper and iron. Highly processed meats are not a healthy choice, but pasture-raised beef is a nutrient powerhouse. This delicious Bolognese sauce can be made for three meals: Courgetti Bolognese, Meaty stuffed peppers and Low-carb cottage pie (see overleaf), so make sure you cook up plenty!

Bolognese sauce

(make double quantities in preparation for Low carb cottage pie or Meaty stuffed peppers)

400g fresh tomatoes
Olive oil, avocado oil or ghee,
    for cooking
2 onions, finely chopped
250g mushrooms, sliced
2 garlic cloves, chopped
2 tsp miso paste
500g best-quality minced
    beef (the best you can get)
2 tsp dried basil
2 tsp dried oregano
2 tbsp tomato purée
2 x 400g tins of
    chopped tomatoes
2 tbsp coconut aminos
Salt and black pepper, to taste

TO SERVE
Courgetti (spiralised courgette)
    or low-carb pasta (see
    page 81)
Grated Cheddar or
    nutritional yeast

1. Preheat the oven to 170°C fan.

2. Lay out your fresh tomatoes on a baking tray, douse in oil or ghee and roast in the oven for 15 minutes.

3. In the meantime, fry the onions, mushrooms and garlic in a large saucepan with a small amount of olive oil or ghee and miso for 5 minutes until the onion and mushrooms soften. Next add the minced beef and cook for a further 10 minutes.

4. Remove the roasted tomatoes from the oven and blend until smooth.

5. Add the dried herbs, blended roasted tomatoes, tomato purée, tinned tomatoes, coconut aminos and salt and pepper to the pan with the beef. Simmer on a low heat for 20 minutes.

6. Serve with either courgetti or low-carb pasta topped with grated cheese or nutritional yeast for a dairy-free cheese flavour plus extra goodness!

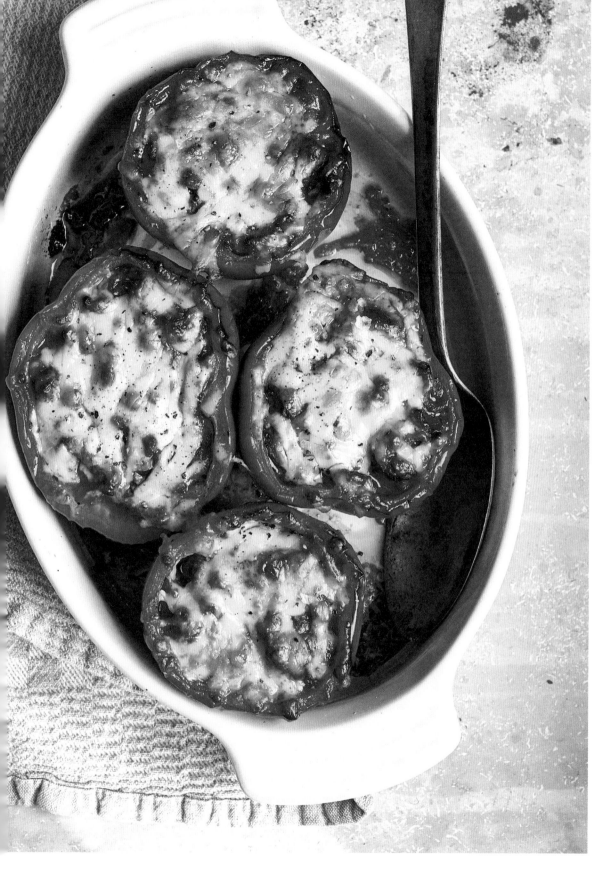

Meaty stuffed peppers

A super simple supper that takes no time to prepare but bursting with flavour.

Serves 2

4 red peppers
Olive oil, for cooking
Bolognese sauce (see page 204)
A handful of goat's Cheddar
    or cow's Cheddar, grated

FOR A DAIRY-FREE VERSION
3 tbsp nutritional yeast
3 tbsp coconut yoghurt
2 tbsp coconut aminos

1. Preheat the oven to 175°C fan.

2. Slice your peppers in half, removing the inner seeds and white centre. Rub the pepper halves in some oil and place on a baking tray.

3. Fill each half with Bolognese sauce. Sprinkle with grated Cheddar or make a dairy-free cheese topping by mixing the nutritional yeast with the coconut yoghurt and coconut aminos before spooning over the meat-filled peppers.

4. Bake for 35 minutes.

(Photographed on page 205)

Low-carb cottage pie

A light and low-carb twist on a family favourite.

1 medium celeriac, peeled
    and cut into cubes
A good knob of goat's butter
    or cow's butter
Bolognese sauce (see page 204)
60g Cheddar, grated,
    or nutritional yeast
Salt and black pepper, to taste

1. Preheat the oven to 175°C fan.

2. Cook the celeriac cubes in a pan of boiling water until soft. Drain, then mash the celeriac cubes by hand or in a blender, adding salt, pepper and some butter for extra richness.

3. Spoon the Bolognese sauce into an ovenproof dish and top with the celeriac mash.

4. Sprinkle with cheese or nutritional yeast before baking for 35–40 minutes or until piping hot.

Frittata ... but not as you know it

Protein not only helps us to feel fuller for longer, it also gives our body the building blocks for making muscle and creating luscious locks and supple skin. This twist on a classic frittata gives you a satisfying crunch and an extra hit of fibre.

1. Preheat the oven to 170°C fan.

2. Wash the chard thoroughly to remove any grit, then separate the stalks from the leaves. Slice the stalks horizontally.

3. Add a spoonful of ghee or butter to an ovenproof frying pan. Add the shallots or onions and chard stalks and fry until softened and slightly golden.

4. In the meantime, beat the eggs together, seasoning with salt and pepper to your liking.

5. Dry and chop the chard leaves and add these and the garlic to the almost-cooked stalks, then cook for a further 4–5 minutes. Drain away any excess moisture before pouring in the beaten eggs.

6. Place the pan in the oven for 5 minutes.

7. Add the bread roll and cheese to a blender or food processor and pulse to create breadcrumbs.

8. Remove the pan from the oven, top with the breadcrumbs and return to the oven for a further 5–10 minutes.

9. Remove from the oven and carefully slice into wedges. Serve each person one wedge crumb-side up and one wedge crumb-side down.

Serve with sauerkraut and Roasted red pepper pesto (see page 152).

200g Swiss chard
Ghee or butter, for frying
2 banana shallots
    or onions, diced
9 eggs
2 garlic cloves, crushed
1 Best bun (see
    page 170), roughly chopped
60g Cheddar, roughly chopped
Salt and black pepper, to taste

MAIN MEALS

Grilled goat's cheese, pea shoots, pomegranate & raspberry vinaigrette

This tart and tangy combo is packed with antioxidants, protein and minerals. Goat's cheese can be swapped for feta or even grilled tofu, for a vegan alternative.

3–4 slices of goat's cheese
    log per person
A handful of pea shoots
    or rocket
100g mixed leaves
Raspberry blush vinaigrette
    (see page 148), for drizzling
A handful of pumpkin seeds
A handful of pecans
A spoonful of
    pomegranate seeds

1. Line a grill rack with foil and place the sliced goat's cheese discs under a hot grill for 3–5 minutes each side until golden.

2. Dress the plates with pea shoots and mixed leaves before adding the grilled goat's cheese discs.

3. Generously douse the leaves and cheese in vinaigrette and sprinkle with pumpkin seeds, pecans and pomegranate seeds to finish.

MAIN MEALS

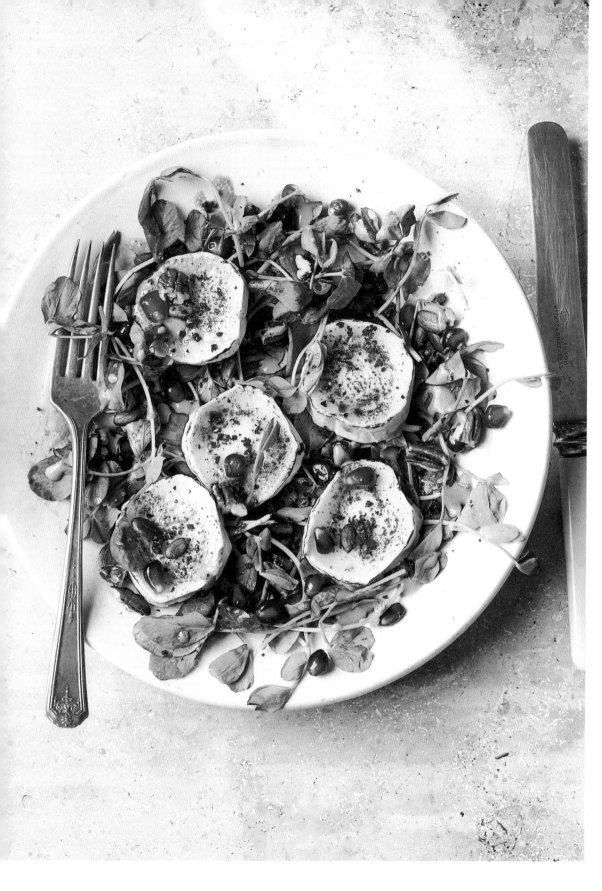

Peanut dipping sauce

This delicious, rich, perfect peanut dipping sauce is so good! Adjust the heat to your taste …

1 tbsp coconut oil
1 small onion, diced
1 tsp chilli flakes
1 tsp crushed or powdered garlic
1 tsp ground coriander
½ tsp ground ginger
    or grated fresh
2 tbsp tomato purée
400ml tin of coconut milk
160g peanut butter
2 tbsp coconut aminos
Juice of 1 lime
A pinch of salt

1. Add the coconut oil to a pan and heat. Add the onion, chilli flakes, garlic, ground coriander and ginger and sauté the onions until they are soft and browned.

2. Add the tomato purée, coconut milk and peanut butter, stirring the mix and combining until smooth.

3. Lastly, remove from the heat and add the coconut aminos, lime juice and salt.

Serve over skewered chicken, skewered veggies or tofu with salad, sauerkraut or Turmeric & coconut cauli-rice (page 144).

MAIN MEALS

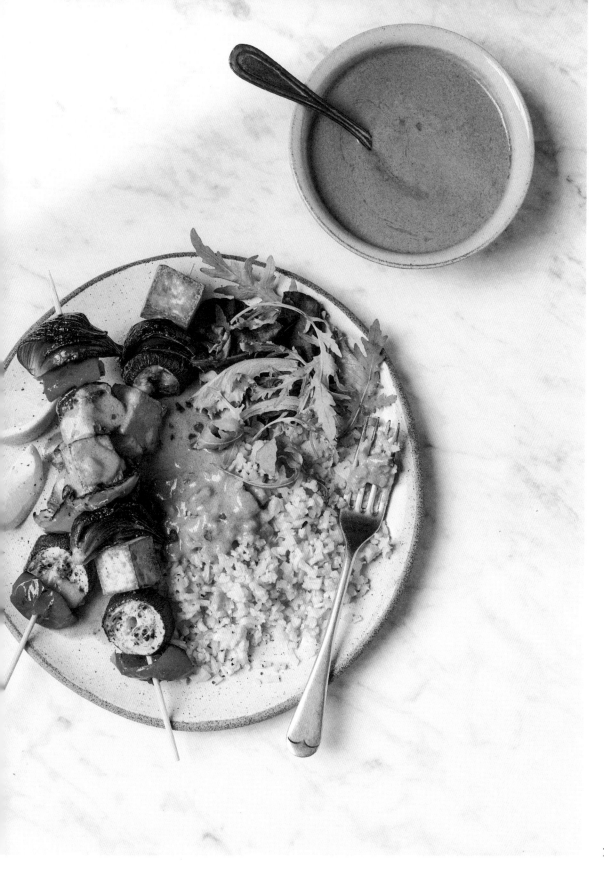

Goat's cheese mousse, balsamic onions, walnuts & Tenderstem broccoli

Prepare the mousse in the morning (it takes minutes!) and whip up the Tenderstem broccoli when you're ready to eat. This mousse is rich in calcium and protein, and kind to your gut, being packed with probiotics and because goat's cheese is easier to digest than cheese made from cow's milk.

Butter, for frying
5 eggs
I round goat's cheese
30ml balsamic vinegar
4 onions, sliced
A handful of walnuts,
     plus extra to serve
200g Tenderstem broccoli
Beetroot salt, to taste

TO SERVE
Sauerkraut and salad leaves
A drizzle of olive oil, to finish

1. Heat a frying pan and add a little butter. In a mixing bowl, add four of the five eggs and beat together before adding to the heated frying pan, then cook, stirring.

2. Chop the goat's cheese into chunks and add to the semi-scrambled egg mix. Continue to cook until the eggs are fully scrambled and the goat's cheese is incorporated. Switch off the heat and allow the eggs to cool a little.

3. Empty the scrambled egg mix into a blender and combine on a high speed until smooth. Add the yolk of the remining egg and continue to blend until fully incorporated.

4. Transfer into two ramekins and refrigerate for 30 minutes. You can leave it in the fridge for up to 3 days.

5. While the mousse chills, add a dollop of butter and the balsamic vinegar to a frying pan on a medium heat. Sauté the onions, stirring occasionally. Reduce the heat to a low setting and add the walnuts. Simmer for a further 15 minutes, stirring occasionally, until dark and sticky.

6. Steam the Tenderstem broccoli for 2–3 minutes.

7. Share the broccoli between two plates, adding the ramekin of goat's cheese mousse to each plate. Spoon the onion and walnut mix over the broccoli and goat's cheese mousse and finish with a few more walnuts and a sprinkle of beetroot salt. Serve with sauerkraut and a few salad leaves. Drizzle with olive oil to finish.

MAIN MEALS

Lemony fish dippers

Fish goujons – the easy way! When you're hungry and in a hurry, this recipe is a saviour.

1. Preheat the oven to 180°C fan.

2. Roughly cut the bread into chunks before adding to a blender and pulsing into breadcrumbs.

3. Take two dishes, and on one lay out the breadcrumbs, on the other dollop the mayonnaise.

4. Slice the fish into goujon-sized pieces, then roll in the mayonnaise, before rolling in the breadcrumbs.

5. Place the coated fish into an ovenproof dish and bake in the oven for 20 minutes until the outside is golden brown.

Serve with a wedge of lemon, sauerkraut, salad leaves and a simple salad of choice – cucumber and cherry tomatoes or Raw slaw or Remoulade (page 154).

1 Best bun (see page 170) or 2 slices of Low-carb loaf (page 174)
40g Lemon olive oil mayonnaise (see page 151)
200–250g salmon or fish of choice

MAIN MEALS

Pumpkin, pesto-crusted salmon

This magnesium-packed fish dish is not only delicious and simple, but also super nutrient dense!

2 salmon fillets, skin on
2 heaped tbsp Lemon olive oil
  mayonnaise (homemade,
  see page 151)
1 Best bun (see page 170) or
  2 slices of Low-carb loaf
  (page 174), roughly chopped
50g goat's Cheddar or
  cow's Cheddar, grated
50g pumpkin seeds
A handful of fresh basil

1. Preheat the oven to 180°C fan.

2. Place the salmon fillets skin side down in an ovenproof dish. Drop a tablespoon of mayonnaise on each fillet and smear evenly over the top the salmon.

3. Add the roughly chopped bread, cheese, pumpkin seeds and basil to a blender and pulse to form chunky breadcrumbs.

4. Pile the breadcrumbs onto the mayo-surface of the salmon. Bake for 15–18 minutes until cooked through.

Serve with a wedge of lemon, steamed broccoli or Broccamoley (page 164) plus a little fresh sauerkraut.

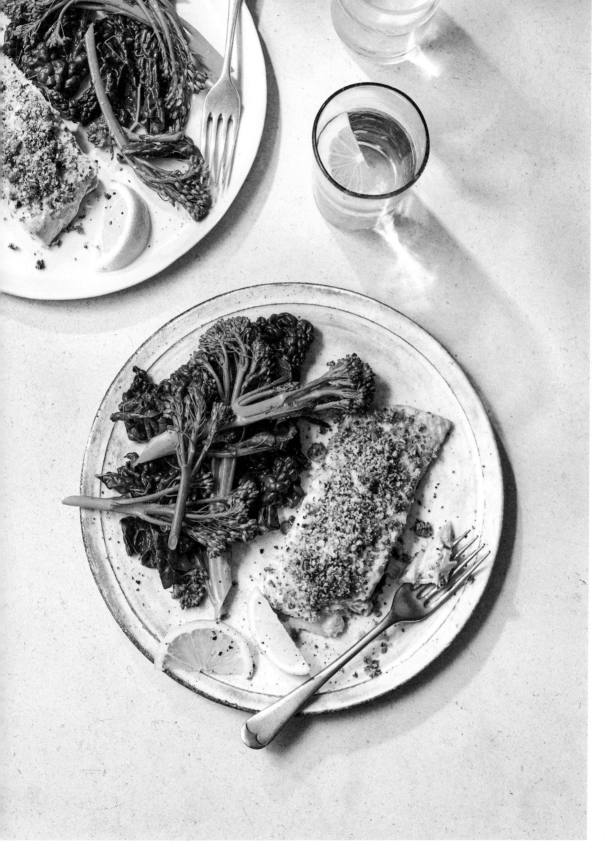

In a hurry curry

This speedy sauce is inspired by the flavours of Kastu curry and is the perfect addition to roast veg, roast chicken or baked fish.

A selection of veggies
    (such as 2–3 courgettes,
    1 red pepper, deseeded,
    1 small celeriac, peeled,
    2–3 small onions,1 small
    butternut squash, peeled
    and deseeded)
2–3 tbsp coconut oil
1 onion, diced
2.5cm chunk of fresh ginger,
    grated or 1 heaped tsp
    ground ginger
1 tbsp ground turmeric
2 tsp mild curry powder
200ml chicken stock, bone
    broth or vegan stock
1 tbsp coconut aminos
200ml coconut milk
1 tbsp tapioca powder
    or flour, to thicken

TO SERVE
300g Turmeric & coconut
    cauli-rice (see page
    144 or store-bought)
Sauerkraut
A handful of chopped
    fresh herbs
A dollop of natural
    or coconut yoghurt

1. Preheat the oven to 180°C fan.

2. Add a selection of chopped veggies to a roasting tin, cover in coconut oil and roast for 40–45 minutes.

3. Fry the diced onion in coconut oil in a frying pan with the spices until soft and golden. Add the stock, coconut aminos and coconut milk and stir through until smooth and well combined. Reduce the heat.

4. In a small bowl whisk together the tapioca powder or flour with 1 tablespoon of water and add to the pan of sauce, stirring until it thickens.

5. Add the selection of roast veggies to the pan. Serve with Turmeric & coconut cauli-rice and sauerkraut. Top with a handful of chopped fresh herbs and a dollop of natural or coconut yoghurt.

Bitter-sweet sesame bok choy salad with salmon

Bitter greens are an excellent support for our liver, as well as being loaded with nutrients. Bitter flavours also help reduce sugar cravings … win-win!

1. Preheat the oven to 170°C fan.

2. Add the coconut oil to a pan on a low heat. When melted, add the coconut aminos, tahini and grated ginger and gently cook for 4–5 minutes, stirring to combine.

3. Place the salmon steaks in an ovenproof dish. Pour half of the tahini and ginger dressing on top of the salmon, ensuring the steaks are well coated. Sprinkle with sesame seeds and bake for 12–14 minutes until cooked through.

4. About 5 minutes before the end of the salmon cooking time, halve or quarter the bok choy. Heat the pan with the remaining tahini and ginger mix and add the bok choy, then sauté for 2–4 minutes.

5. Serve the bok choy with the salmon steaks and some kimchi or sauerkraut.

2 tbsp coconut oil
1 tbsp coconut aminos
2 tsp black or white tahini paste
A 2.5cm chunk of
    fresh ginger, grated
2 salmon steaks
2 tbsp sesame seeds
3–4 bok choy
Kimchi or sauerkraut,
    to serve

MAIN MEALS

Beetroot & goat's cheese cauli-rice risotto

Absolutely delicious … packed with goodness and certain to keep you feeling full and satisfied!

6–10 beetroots, roughly chopped (make more for a Double beetroot salad for the next day, see page 200), or raw
Coconut oil, for roasting
1 white onion or 3 spring onions, diced
1 garlic clove, minced
400g cauli-rice (plain, raw Cauli-rice, see page 143, or store-bought)
150ml veggie stock or 4–5 ice cubes of Bone broth or 150ml of fresh bone broth
1 tsp beetroot salt, plus extra to serve
A log of goat's cheese, sliced
Drizzle of Raspberry blush vinaigrette (optional, see page 148)
A handful of sunflower seeds and pumpkin seeds
Chopped fresh herbs of choice

1. Preheat the oven to 180°C fan.

2. Roughly chop the beetroot, coating them in coconut oil, then roast for 40 minutes or until soft.

3. Add a little coconut oil into a large pan and sauté the onions and garlic until soft and brown. Add in the cauli-rice and roasted beetroot.

4. Add in the veggie stock or bone broth and combine.

5. Take half of the beetroot-cauli mix, add to a blender and combine until smooth.

6. Reintroduce the smooth mix back into the remaining half of the beetroot-cauli mix and stir. Add in the 1 teaspoon of beetroot salt.

7. In the meantime, place the sliced goat's cheese discs on a sheet of tin foil under a hot grill for 2–3 minutes before turning and browning on both sides.

8. Plate up the cauli-rice risotto, placing on top the grilled goat's cheese discs, drizzling with Raspberry blush vinaigrette, topping with a handful of seeds, chopped fresh herbs and a sprinkle of beetroot salt.

For a vegan option, add a few dollops of coconut yoghurt instead of the goat's cheese.

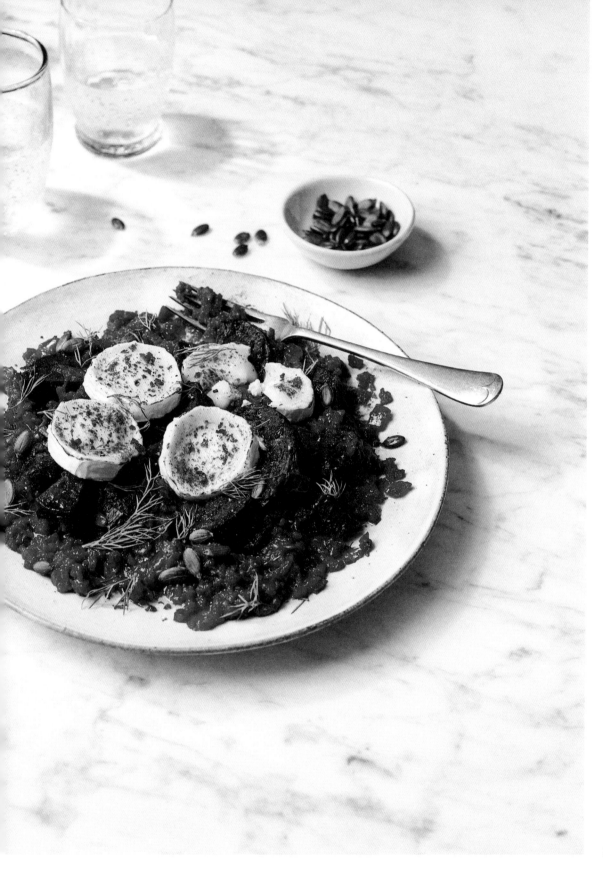

Keto-friendly chicken

When you're looking for a healthier version of a takeaway classic, this low-carb chicken is super tasty.

2 boneless chicken breasts
2 eggs
20g coconut flour
180g ground almonds
1 tsp smoked paprika
1 tsp salt
1 tsp garlic powder
½ tsp ground coriander
½ tsp ground cumin
Black pepper, to taste

1. Preheat the oven to 180°C fan. Line a baking tray with parchment paper.

2. Slice the chicken breasts into the desired thickness. Crack the eggs into a bowl and beat until combined.

3. In another bowl, combine the coconut flour, ground almonds and spices. Rub the mix together with your fingertips until fine in texture and lump-free.

4. Dip the chicken strips into the egg mix, then into the flour mix, before placing onto the lined baking tray.

5. Bake in the oven for 15–20 minutes until cooked through and golden.

Serve with crispy lettuce, chopped cucumber salad, Lemon olive oil mayonnaise (see page 151) and sauerkraut.

MAIN MEALS

Desserts + Snacks

Sweet potato brownies

Packed with fibre and antioxidants and deliciously moreish, these sweet potato brownies can be eaten warm, cold – even frozen!

500g roasted, unpeeled, cubed sweet potato (weigh after it's cooked not before as it loses weight during cooking)
120g coconut oil, melted
170g almond flour
50g erythritol or 50ml maple syrup
100g cacao powder
1 tsp baking powder
A handful of pecans or walnuts
A handful of flaked almonds
Dollop of Blueberry and lime chia jam (see page 135) and a little coconut yoghurt, to serve

1. Preheat the oven to 170°C fan and line a standard-sized brownie tray.

2. Add the warm roasted sweet potato and melted coconut oil to a food processor and combine on high power until smooth. Transfer to a mixing bowl.

3. Add the almond flour, erythritol or maple syrup, cacao powder and baking powder to the sweet potato mix.

4. Add the chopped nuts and transfer to the lined brownie tray. Top with the flaked almonds.

5. Bake for 15 minutes, then allow to cool before slicing.

6. Serve with a dollop of blueberry and lime chia jam and a little coconut yoghurt.

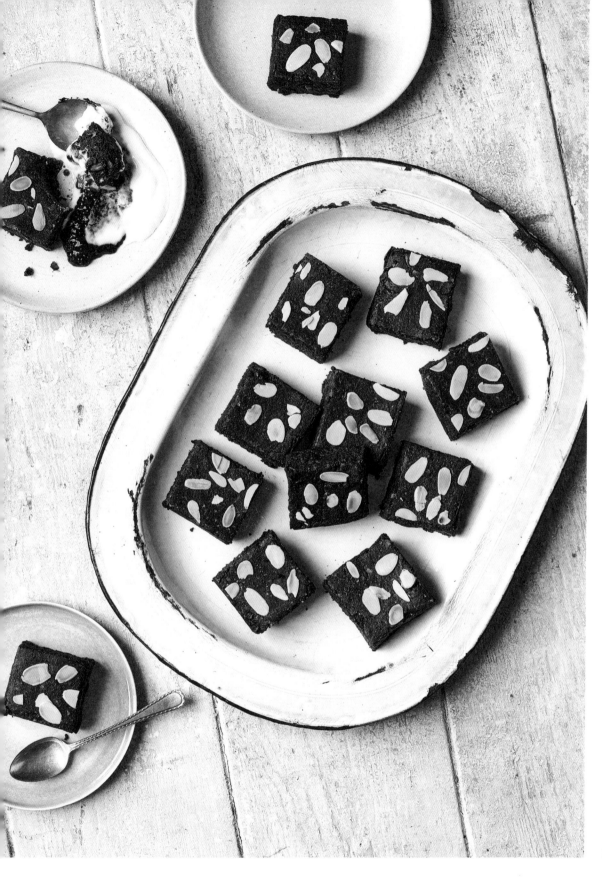

Carrot & apple muffins

These muffins are naturally sweetened by the grated carrot, apple and cinnamon. This fibre-fest will keep you feeling full and satisfied without a blood-sugar spike.

90g coconut oil, melted, plus extra for greasing
5 eggs
375g ground almonds
150g sultanas
90g walnuts or pecans, roughly chopped, plus a few extra to serve
3 tsp baking powder
3 tsp ground cinnamon
1 tsp salt
375g carrots, grated
375g apples, grated (green apples for a lower carb content)
Zest and juice of 1 unwaxed lemon
Coconut or natural yoghurt, to serve

1. Preheat the oven to 170°C fan and grease a 12-hole muffin tin.

2. In a mixing bowl, beat the eggs and combine with the melted coconut oil.

3. Add the ground almonds, sultanas, walnuts or pecans, baking powder, cinnamon and salt to the liquid egg mix, along with the grated carrots and apples and mix together to form a thick batter. Add in a quarter of the lemon juice (use the rest in drinking water) and half of the lemon zest.

4. Spoon the thick mix into your greased muffin tray. Bake for 22–25 minutes. Remove from the oven and leave to cool.

5. Serve with a dollop of coconut or natural yoghurt, a pecan or a walnut and sprinkle with the remaining lemon zest.

These muffins freeze really well for up to 3 months, making batch cooking so much easier!

DESSERTS + SNACKS

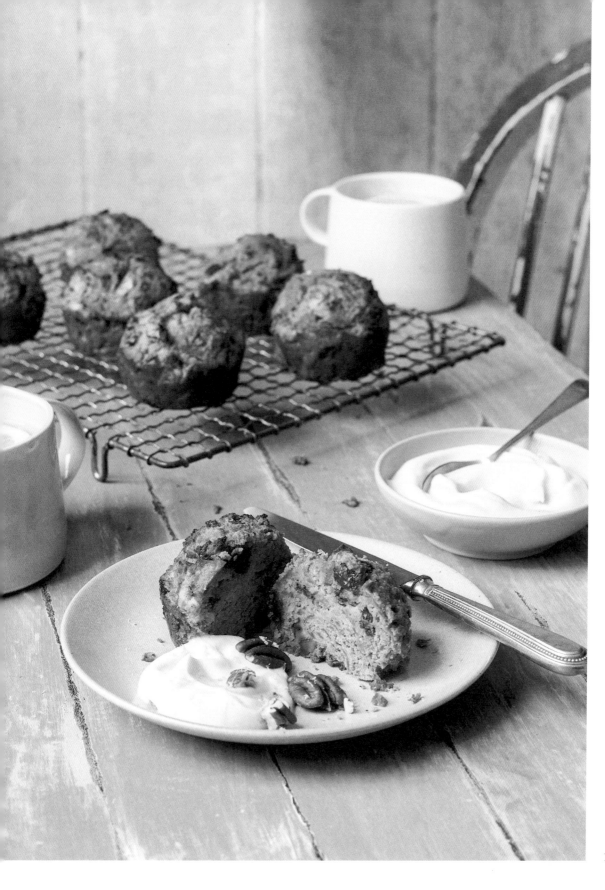

Chia chocolate-raspberry pudding

Chia is a super source of calcium, a great fibre fix and an excellent dose of plant-based omega-3 fatty acids. Chia also gives a wonderful gelatinous texture to desserts.

I ripe avocado, peeled
    and stoned
300ml unsweetened nut milk
4 tbsp cacao powder
100g frozen or fresh raspberries
A pinch of salt
I tsp ground cinnamon
I tbsp raw honey or
    erythritol (optional)
4 tbsp chia seeds

TO SERVE
Natural yoghurt, extra berries,
    a sprinkle of cacao powder
    or dark chocolate shavings

1. In a blender, add the avocado flesh, nut milk, cacao, raspberries, pinch of salt, cinnamon and sweetener, if using, then blend until smooth.

2. Stir in the chia seeds.

3. Pour the mix into two ramekins and refrigerate for 30 minutes or until set.

4. Top with a dollop of natural yoghurt, extra berries and a sprinkle of cacao or dark chocolate shavings.

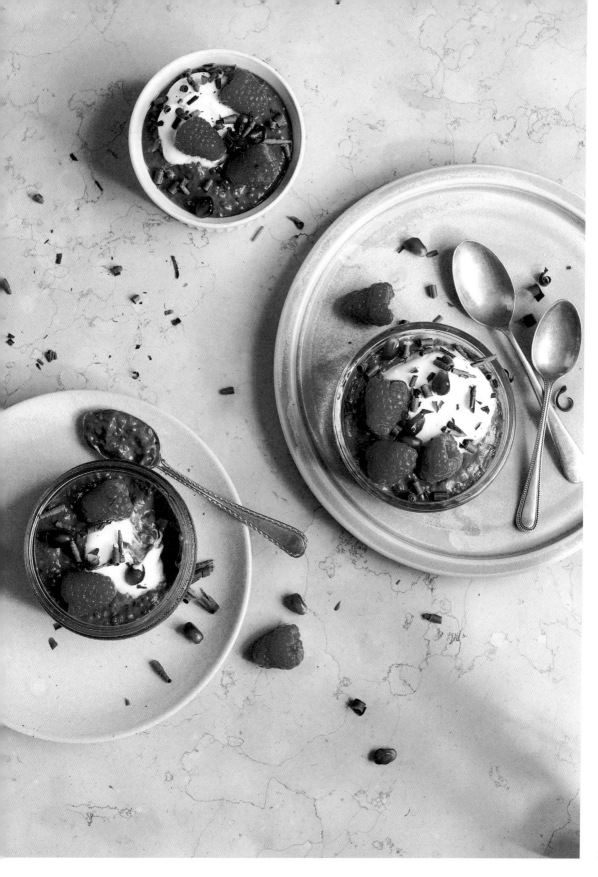

Lemon, passion fruit & pistachio cheesecake pots

This speedy cheesecake is best served in ramekin pots. The passion fruit and lemon combo offers a heady mix of zest and passion fruit punch! For a speedy version, leave out the base and top with a few crunchy nuts or a handful of blended Grain-no-la.

40g butter or coconut oil
80g Grain-no-la (see page 133)
    or store-bought keto
    granola (see page 81)
150g ricotta cheese
3 egg yolks
1–2 tbsp powdered
    erythritol or raw honey
    (or more if needed)
Juice and zest of 1 large
    unwaxed lemon
3 passion fruits
100ml double cream
1 tsp gelatin (Planet Paleo
    do a high-quality gelatin)
A handful of Nutfix &
    chill (see page 240) or
    pistachio nuts

DESSERTS + SNACKS

1. Melt the butter or coconut oil.

2. Blend the Grain-no-la in a blender to a fine crumb. In a small bowl, combine the Grain-no-la crumbs and melted butter or oil.

3. Spoon the mix between two ramekins and gently press into the base using a spoon (not too hard or the base becomes too compact). Refrigerate while you prepare the filling.

4. In a blender, combine the ricotta cheese, egg yolks, sweetener, lemon juice and half of the zest until smooth. Mix in the seeds from two passion fruit.

5. In a small pan, gently heat the cream and melt the gelatin until fully dissolved and fully incorporated (6–10 minutes).

6. Mix the gelatin-cream in with the blended ricotta mix. Pour onto the cheesecake bases and refrigerate for 2 hours to set.

7. Top with the remaining passion fruit seeds and the remaining lemon zest before serving. Finish with a few Nutfix & Chill or shelled pistachio nuts.

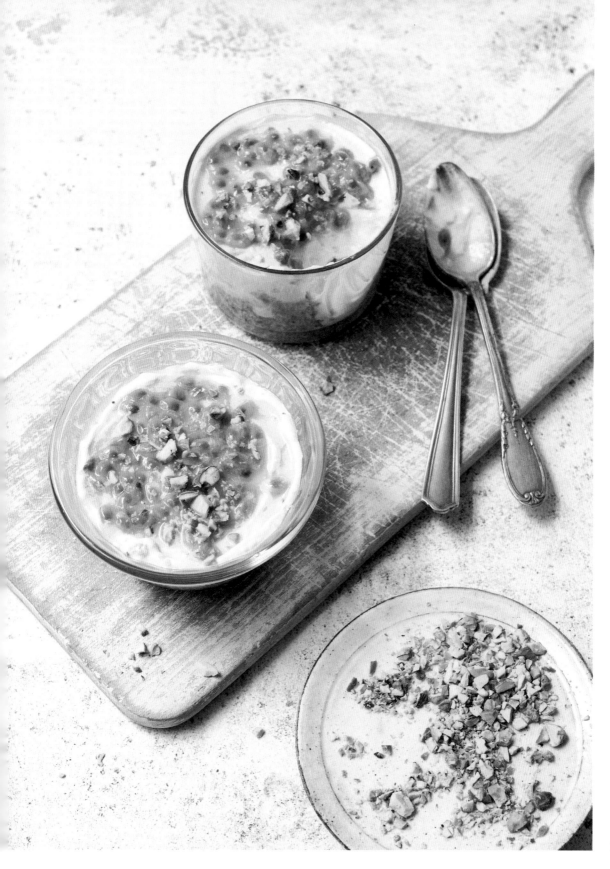

Mini Victoria sponges

Low-carb cake – because life wouldn't be the same without a sponge cake!

110g softened butter, plus
    extra for greasing
80g granulated erythritol
180g cream cheese
7 large eggs
230g ground almonds
½ tsp pink Himalayan salt
1 tsp of gluten-free
    baking powder

FILLING
200ml double cream
Raspberry or Blueberry
    chia jam (see page 134)
Powdered erythritol, to dust

1. Preheat the oven to 170°C fan. Grease a 6-case mini-cake silicon mould tray.

2. Beat the erythritol and butter together until pale and fluffy before adding the cream cheese and continuing to beat.

3. Crack the eggs into a separate bowl, beating together before adding to the creamed butter mix. Combine thoroughly.

4. Add the ground almonds, salt and baking powder and combine into a smooth cake batter. Fill the silicon mould with the cake batter and bake for 20 minutes. Remove from the oven and allow to cool.

5. Whip up the double cream until stiff, but not overwhipped. Slice the cooled cakes through the centre and add a dollop of cream (or pipe on top for a more polished finish!) Add a dollop of jam and replace the sponge top before dusting with powdered erythritol.

VARIATION
For a variation on this cake, add cinnamon and allspice to the sponge and serve with stewed apples and piped cream.

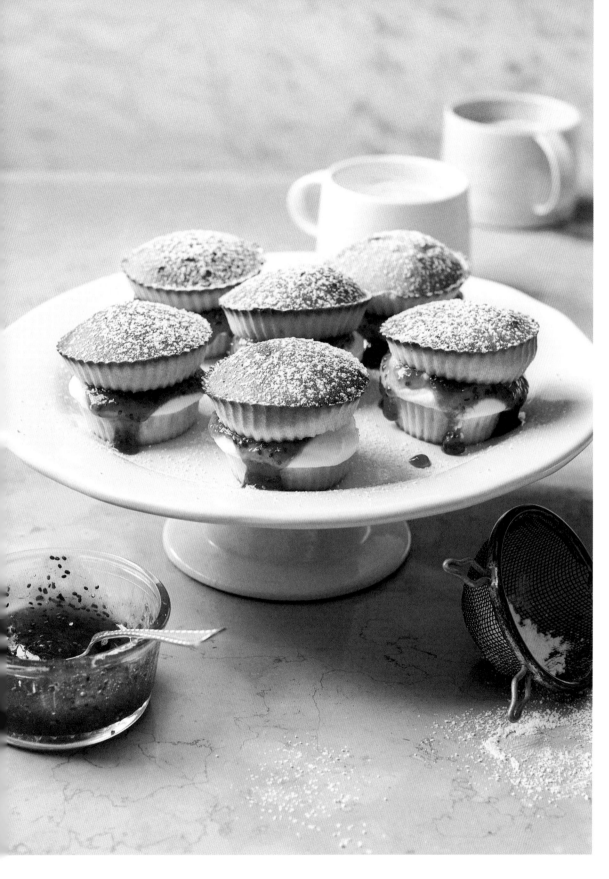

Strawberry chocolate miso mousse

This mousse takes minutes to make and really helps to satisfy a sweet craving without sending blood sugars rocketing!

1 large ripe avocado, peeled and stoned
A few handfuls of strawberries, plus 2 to decorate
1 tsp miso paste
4 heaped tbsp cacao powder, plus extra for dusting
2 dollops of natural or coconut yoghurt (vanilla Cocos Organic works well!)

1. Add the flesh of the avocado, the strawberries, miso and cacao powder to a blender and combine until smooth and creamy.

2. Spoon into two ramekins, adding a dollop of natural or coconut yoghurt. Top each with a whole strawberry and dust with cacao powder to finish.

3. Refrigerate for up to 3 days or until needed, or eat straight away!

For extra goodness, add a tablespoon of collagen peptides and/or sprinkle with Nutfix & Chill (see page 250).

DESSERTS + SNACKS

Fruit & nut shortbreads

This recipe can be adapted to add less sweetness, or you can add some zing to the base with orange oil or peppermint oil to make a chocolate orange biscuit. Let your imagination go wild!

1. Preheat the oven to 170°C fan.

2. Add the coconut oil to a saucepan to gently melt.

3. Create a golden linseed flour by whizzing the golden linseeds in a blender before adding to a mixing bowl. Repeat the process for the sunflower seeds and add to the same mixing bowl.

4. Pulse the flaked almonds in a blender to create a chopped, confetti-like consistency and add to the mixing bowl.

5. Add all the remaining ingredients, and the melted coconut oil, to the mixing bowl and combine well.

6. Grease a wide-based muffin tray (ideally you want to use silicon moulds because these biscuits pop out beautifully when they're chilled). Fill your greased moulds halfway with the biscuit mix and press down using the back of a spoon until it is flat and level.

7. Bake for 14–18 minutes before removing from the oven and allowing to cool.

8. In the meantime, gently melt the dark chocolate, then spoon over the cooled biscuit bases to create an approximately 5mm thick layer of chocolate.

9. While the chocolate is still wet, sprinkle chopped nuts, seeds and the optional dried fruit of choice onto the chocolate topping. Store in the fridge and use with 7 days, or freeze and use within 3 months.

340g coconut oil, plus extra
   for greasing
150g linseeds
200g sunflower seeds
100g almond flakes
250g almond flour
150g desiccated coconut
1 tsp salt
120g erythritol

TO TOP IT OFF
90g bar of dark
   chocolate of choice
Chopped mixed nuts
   – pistachios, pecans,
   walnuts, almonds
A handful of pumpkin seeds
Golden sultanas or dried
   cranberries (optional)

DESSERTS + SNACKS

Mint-choc shortbreads

A delicious, low-carb, buttery shortbread, perfect for a light dessert or an after-dinner treat.

200g ground almonds
6 tbsp melted butter
50g erythritol
100g dark chocolate,
    broken into squares
¼ tsp peppermint extract
A handful of finely chopped
    hazelnuts or pecans

1. Combine the ground almonds, melted butter and erythritol in a mixing bowl to create a dough. Wrap in cling film and chill in the fridge for 30 minutes.

2. Preheat the oven to 165°C fan.

3. Between two sheets of parchment paper, roll the biscuit dough until it's approximately 1¼cm in thickness.

4. Using a sharp knife, cut into 10 rectangular-shaped biscuits and then, using a fork, prick a few holes into each.

5. Transfer to a lined baking tray and bake for 12 minutes. Remove from the oven and allow to cool.

6. Gently melt the chocolate in a heatproof bowl set over a pan of boiling water, but not touching the water below, and add the peppermint extract. Once melted, remove the bowl from the pan and dunk each cooled shortbread into the melted mint chocolate, coating three-quarters of the biscuit.

7. Set onto a sheet of parchment paper, sprinkle with the chopped nuts and refrigerate to set for 15 minutes in the fridge.

VARIATION
For variation, use orange extract with pistachio nuts or dark chocolate with a few freeze-dried raspberries sprinkled on top.

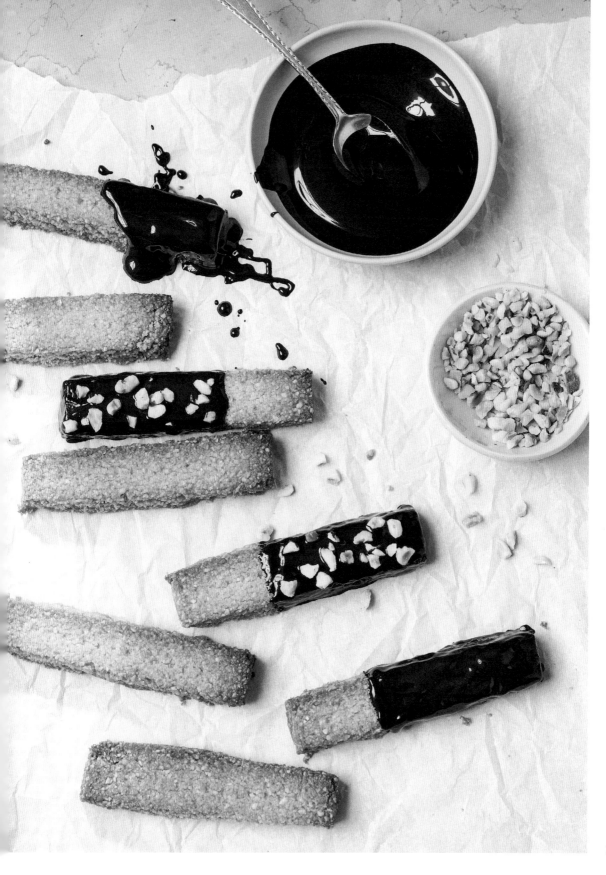

Toasted teacake with Roquefort

The combination of a delicious, creamy Roquefort and warm, spiced teacake works a treat for this speedy snack. Roquefort, known as 'The King of Cheese' in France, is traditionally made with unpasturised sheep's milk and aged in caves near Toulouse, giving it a distinctive tangy flavour.

I Glazed low-carb teacake
    (page 173)
40g Roquefort cheese

I. Slice the teacake in half and grill until it is golden brown on both sides. Slice up the Roquefort and serve on the hot, toasted teacake. Simple … but delicious!

ALTERNATIVE TOPPINGS
A tasty alternative to Roquefort is to add nut butters to your toasted teacake – crunchy almond butter, macadamia nut butter – or a simple peanut butter will work well, with a sprinkle of sea salt. Wonderful!

A slice of goat's cheese on top of your toasted teacake is another really tasty option. Grill until the cheese is golden brown and gooey. Top with a few fresh raspberries to add an extra tang of berry goodness.

DESSERTS + SNACKS

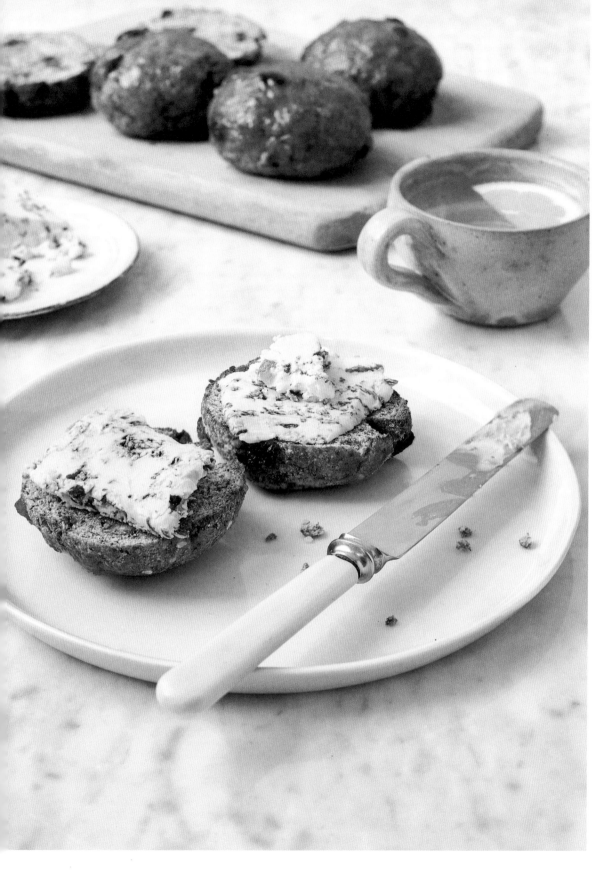

Lemon & poppy seed muffins

These zingy lemon muffins are packed with protein and fibre as well as being low in sugar. They freeze well and are ideal for batch-cooking!

Coconut oil or butter,
    for greasing
390g ground almonds
4 tsp gluten-free baking powder
120g erythritol
3 eggs, beaten
300g soured cream or
    coconut cream for
    a dairy-free version
1½ tsp vanilla extract
1½ tbsp poppy seeds
150ml unsweetened nut
    milk of choice
Juice and zest of
    1 unwaxed lemon
100ml double cream

1. Preheat the oven to 170°C fan and grease a 12-case muffin tray with coconut oil or butter.

2. Combine all of the ingredients except the cream, and using half the lemon zest, in a large mixing bowl.

3. Pour the muffin mix equally into the greased muffin holes and bake in the oven for 20–25 minutes until golden and well risen. Remove from the oven and allow to cool on a wire rack.

4. Whip the double cream by hand or using a whisk. Pipe the double cream onto the cooled muffins and sprinkle with the remaining lemon zest.

Erythritol is used to sweeten these muffins, making them super low in carbs. Erythritol is a sugar alcohol that doesn't raise blood sugar levels in the same way that cane sugar does, but provides the satisfying sweetness allowing you to have your cake and eat it!

Cheese discs

Perfect for when you fancy something crunchy and a carrot just won't do! These little saviours will take you to cheese heaven …

1. Preheat the oven to 180°C fan.

2. Take an ovenproof dish and line with parchment paper.

3. Using a cookie cutter as a guide, place the cutter on the parchment paper and spoon in 1 heaped tbsp of grated cheese to cover the shape on the paper. Remove the cutter, leaving behind a circle of grated cheese. Repeat until all cheese is used and you have a baking tray of grated cheese discs spaced 2½cm apart.

4. Place the grated cheese discs into the oven for 6–8 minutes. The cheese will bubble, however be careful not to overcook it or let it turn brown.

5. Remove from the oven and allow to cool.

These cheese discs are delicious topped on salads or eaten as a tasty snack.

100g Cheddar (cow or goat's), grated

DESSERTS + SNACKS

239

Nutfix & chill

A rich, sticky, toffee-like medley of nuts. Perfect for a crunchy snack or for topping a yoghurt and berry bowl.

A generous knob of butter
50ml balsamic vinegar
50g almonds
50g pecans
50g walnuts
2 tsp salt

1. Add a knob of butter to a frying pan. Once melted, add the balsamic vinegar and all the nuts, stirring to coat, then on a low heat, allow to simmer gently for 15–20 minutes, stirring occasionally to make sure all the nuts are coated.

2. Once the mix cooks down to a sticky consistency, transfer to parchment paper, sprinkle with salt and allow to cool.

3. Store in a sealed container in the fridge and use within 5 days.

The balsamic vinegar used makes a difference to this recipe ... you want a rich, sticky-toffee end product. The best results I've had with this are with Willy's Live Apple Balsamic Vinegar.

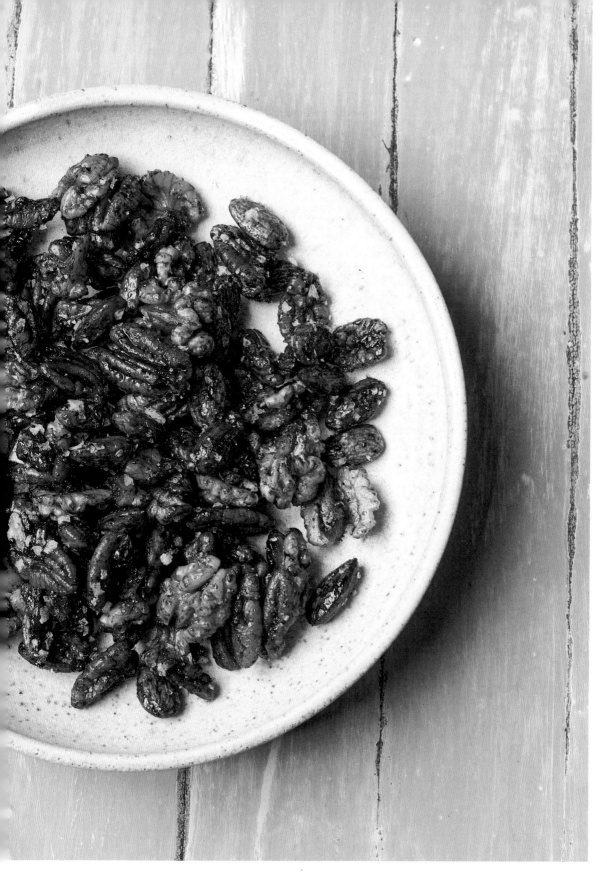

Apple & cinnamon n-oat bars

Fruits of the forest bark

These n-oat bars are the ideal snack to make while making your breakfast! Use the recipe for N-oatmal and simply eat one portion and use the other portion to make these tasty n-oat bars.

Apple-spiced n-oatmeal and cinnamon n-oatmeal (see page 136) or Blueberry & lime n-oatmeal (see page 134)
2 eggs
A handful of nuts and seeds of choice – chopped pecans or hazelnuts, pumpkin or sunflower seeds
Blueberry & lime chia jam (see page 134 – if using blueberry & lime n-oatmeal)

A delicious, fruity, crunchy, low-carb dessert that will satisfy your sweet tooth while packing a punch of nutrients.

400g full-fat natural or vanilla coconut yoghurt
1 tbsp raw honey
1 tbsp light tahini paste
A handful of strawberries, quartered
A handful of blueberries
A handful of macadamia nuts
A sprinkle of coconut flakes
A sprinkle of pumpkin seeds

1. Preheat the oven to 175°C fan.

2. Add the N-Oatmeal to a mixing bowl.

3. Crack in the eggs and add a handful of nuts and seeds of choice. If you want some blueberry and lime flavouring, add two dollops of the chia jam and swirl into the mix.

4. Pour the mix into a square silicon baking mould or square 20cm lined tin, then bake for 30 minutes.

5. Remove from the oven, then cool in the tin before slicing.

1. Line a square 20cm brownie tray with parchment paper.

2. Combine the yoghurt with the honey and tahini. Pour into the lined tray.

3. Lay the strawberry quarters into the yoghurt mix. Sprinkle in the blueberries around the strawberries.

4. Add the macadamia nuts, coconut flakes and pumpkin seeds, then transfer to the freezer for 1 hour or until firm.

5. Lift from the tray using the parchment paper. Snap off sections or, using a sharp knife, cut the bark into squares.

(Photographed opposite)

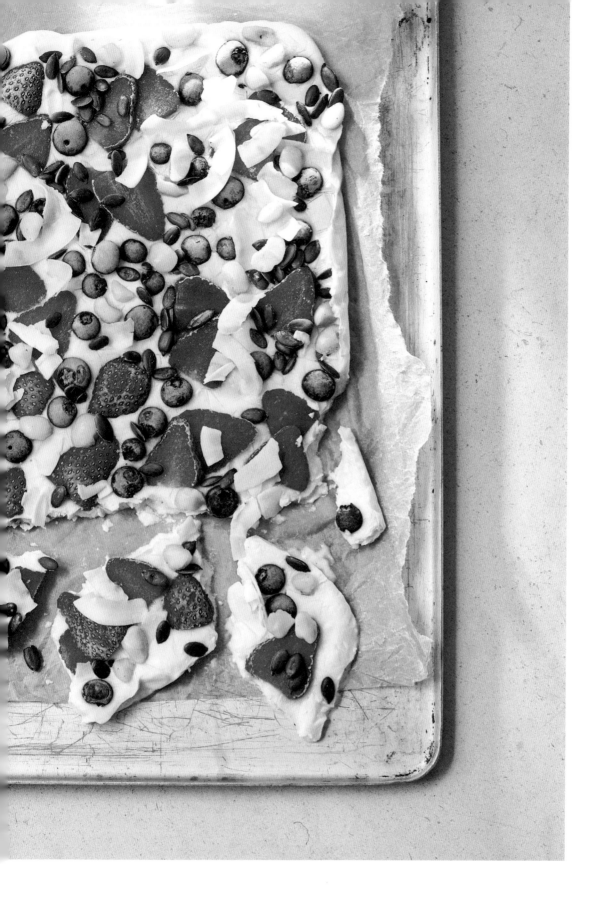

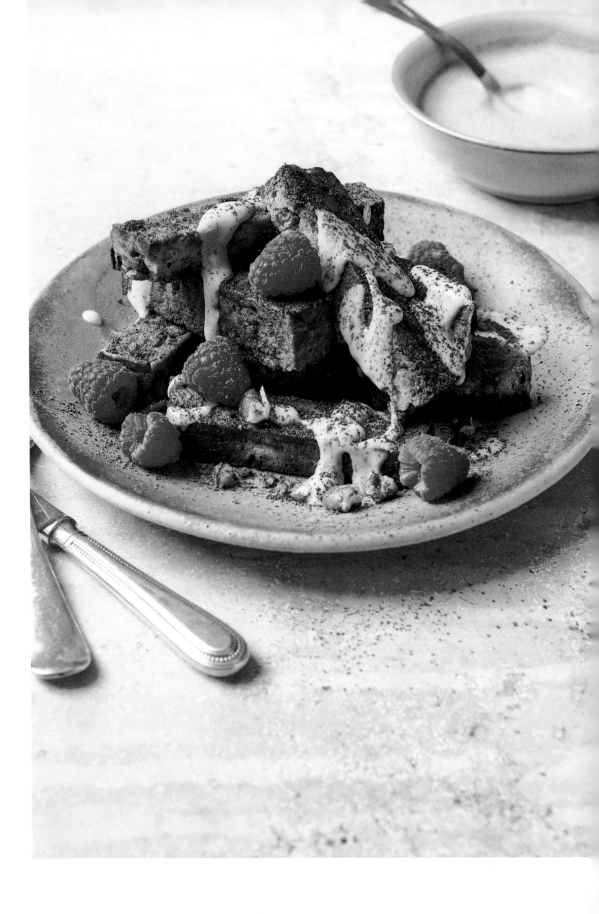

Grilled chocolate, banana & pecan loaf

Having a Banana and crunchy pecan loaf (see page 131) in the fridge is SO handy when you fancy a little something sweet. This recipe uses the loaf to create a delicious dessert in minutes.

1 slice of Banana and crunchy pecan loaf (see page 131)
2 squares of dark chocolate (90% cocoa solids)
A dollop of coconut or natural yoghurt
A few raspberries or blueberries
A handful of chopped pecans

1. Grill the slice of banana bread. Turn it over and top the uncooked side with the dark chocolate, then set under the grill until the chocolate has melted and is spreadable.

2. Top the grilled bread with a dollop of coconut or natural yoghurt, a few fresh raspberries or blueberries and a few chopped pecans.

Fried chocolate fingers

This recipe uses the Banana and crunchy pecan loaf on page 131 as a simple and healthy base for a speedy and nutritious dessert.

A knob of butter or coconut oil
1 tsp ground cinnamon
1–2 slices of Banana and crunchy pecan loaf (see page 131)
2 tbsp natural or vanilla coconut yoghurt
1 tbsp nut butter (pecan nut butter works so well!)
1 tsp cacao powder
½ tsp salt
A handful of chopped pecans
A few berries of choice (optional)

1. Heat a frying pan and add the knob of butter or coconut oil and the cinnamon.

2. Cut the banana loaf slice(s) into chunky fingers and add to the hot melted cinnamon butter in the pan. Allow to gently fry on each side until golden brown.

3. In a mixing bowl, combine the yoghurt and nut butter until smooth and creamy.

4. Stack the cooked fingers in a tower arrangement, dollop over the nut-butter yoghurt and sprinkle with cacao powder, salt and chopped pecans (and a few raspberries or other berries, if you fancy).

(Photographed opposite)

DESSERTS + SNACKS

Chocolate mousse in minutes

This protein-rich mousse is so simple, rich and delicious, it's the perfect craving-buster! The darker the chocolate, the better – aim for 80% cocoa solids and over, easing yourself into the darker side.

Butter, for frying
4 eggs
100g dark chocolate, 80% cocoa
    solids (buttons or pieces)
50ml cream or unsweetened
    nut milk
A handful of chopped pecans
A few raspberries

1. Heat a frying pan and add a little butter. In a mixing bowl, add three of the eggs and the yolk of the fourth egg (you can freeze the leftover egg white). Beat together, add to the heated frying pan and cook until the eggs are scrambled.

2. Gently melt the chocolate in a heatproof bowl set over a pan of boiling water, but not touching the water below. Once melted, remove from the heat and allow to cool slightly.

3. Add the cream or milk to a blender, followed by the scrambled eggs, and blend on a high speed until a smooth, creamy mixture appears.

4. Turn down the speed to a lower setting and slowly pour in the melted chocolate.

5. Transfer the mix to two ramekins and refrigerate for 1 hour. Top with chopped pecans and a few raspberries.

Resources

PRODUCTS & SPECIALITY LOW CARB FOODS

For a range of low-carb products and high-quality supplements
www.sowandarrow.com

FOR MORE INFORMATION

Online
www.paulinecox.com
www.sowandarrow.com
www.dietdoctor.com

Instagram
@paulinejcox

Books
Primal Fat Burner: Nora Gedgaudas
Primal Body, Primal Mind: Nora Gedgaudas
Wheat Belly: Dr William Davis
Why We Get Sick: Benjamin Bikman
Grain Brain: David Perlmutter
The Metabolic Approach to Cancer: Dr Nasha Winters
    and Jess Higgins Kelley
Mind Over Medicine: Dr Lissa Rankin
Breath, The New Science of a Lost Art: James Nester
The Circadian Code: Dr Satchin Panda
The Oxygen Advantage: Patrick McKeown
Walk Yourself Happy: Julia Bradbury

Facebook Groups
Healthy Keto & Low Carb Community

Podcasts
UK Low Carb: Dan Greef
Huberman Lab: Andrew Huberman
The Doctor's Farmacy: Dr Mark Hyman
The Doctor's Kitchen: Dr Rupy Aujla
Feel Better, Live More: Dr Rangan Chatterjee

Communities
Public Health Collaboration: www.phcuk.org

Index

Recipes are in *italics*

Acknowledgements

It is with deep gratitude that I wish to thank all of those who have supported and worked so hard on producing this book.

My superb agent, Rob Shreeve, whose unwavering belief in my work is truly humbling. Editors Lucinda Humphrey and Lizzy Gray, who have championed this book from its earliest conception! Julia Bradbury for her wonderful foreword and words of wisdom. The Nation Centre of Integrative Medicine for their work in furthering our understanding of preventative and optimal healthcare. My husband, Gary Lewis, for his patience and many school pick-ups, my parents for their constant encouragement and my beautiful children. A special thanks to Sam Goodger, store manager at Sow & Arrow, who helps me spin so many plates! Camille Abrahams … my dear close friend and confidante and Savio Joanes … who has helped me in more ways than I could ever acknowledge.

About the Author

Pauline Cox is a Functional Nutritionist with more than twenty years' experience working in health care. Having first trained in Physiotherapy, she went on to gain a Masters in Nutrition, Physical Activity and Public Health and a further Masters level in Integrative Medicine. Pauline frequently appears as a speaker at conferences, events and private engagements. She is the author of *Primal Living in a Modern World* and the co-founder of high street and online low-carb specialists, Sow & Arrow www.sowandarrow.com.

You can find Pauline's blog and contact details at www.paulinecox.com and follow her on Instagram @paulinejcox or join her Facebook group, Healthy Keto & Low Carb Community.

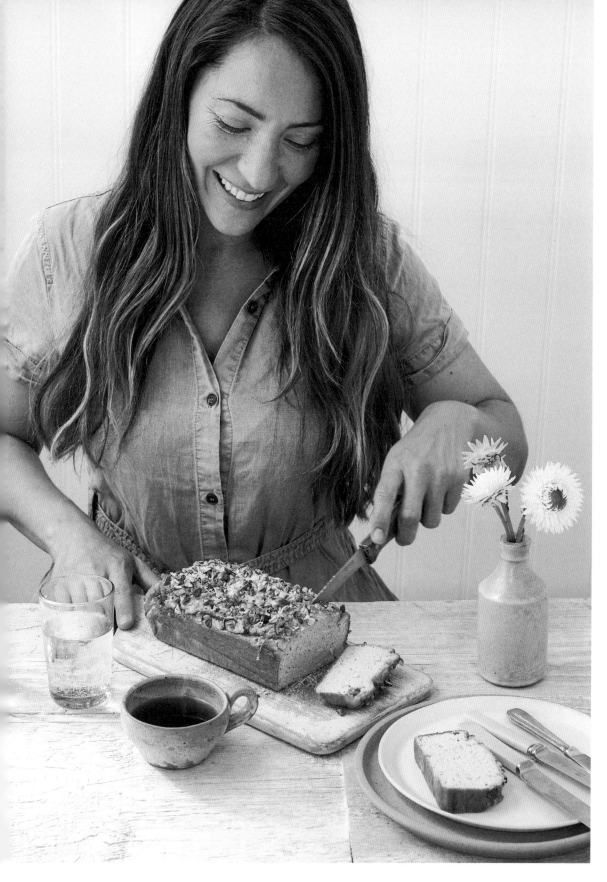

3

Ebury Press an imprint of Ebury Publishing,
20 Vauxhall Bridge Road,
London SW1V 2SA

Ebury Press is part of the Penguin Random House group of companies
whose addresses can be found at global.penguinrandomhouse.com

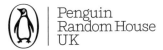

Copyright © Pauline Cox 2023
Photography © Luke Albert 2023
Design by Studio Polka

Pauline Cox has asserted her right to be identified as the author of this
Work in accordance with the Copyright, Designs and Patents Act 1988

First published by Ebury Press in 2023

www.penguin.co.uk

A CIP catalogue record for this book is available from the British Library

ISBN 9781529199109

Colour origination by Altaimage Ltd
Printed and bound in Italy by Lego S.p.A.

The authorised representative in the EEA is Penguin Random House Ireland,
Morrison Chambers, 32 Nassau Street, Dublin D02 YH68

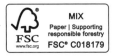

Penguin Random House is committed to a
sustainable future for our business, our readers
and our planet. This book is made from Forest
Stewardship Council® certified paper.